Manual of Ca~~t~~
Surgery

Manual of Cataract Surgery

Second Edition

Edited by

Gavin G. Bahadur, M.D.

Cataract and Anterior Segment Surgeon, The Sinskey Eye Institute, Santa Monica, California; Active Staff, Department of Ophthalmology, St. John's Hospital and Medical Center, Santa Monica

Robert M. Sinskey, M.D.

Clinical Professor of Ophthalmology, Jules Stein Eye Institute, University of California, Los Angeles, UCLA School of Medicine; Active Staff, Department of Ophthalmology, St. John's Hospital and Medical Center, Santa Monica, California

Foreword by

I. Howard Fine, M.D.

Clinical Associate Professor of Ophthalmology, Oregon Health Sciences University School of Medicine, Portland; Co-Founder and Surgeon, Oregon Eye Surgery Center, Oregon Eye Institute, Eugene

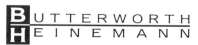

BUTTERWORTH
HEINEMANN

Boston   Oxford   Auckland   Johannesburg   Melbourne   New Delhi

Butterworth–Heinemann supports the efforts of American Forests and the Global ReLeaf program in its campaign for the betterment of trees, forests, and our environment.

Library of Congress Cataloging-in-Publication Data

Bahadur, Gavin G.
    Manual of cataract surgery / Gavin G. Bahadur, Robert M. Sinskey ;
foreword by I. Howard Fine. -- 2nd ed.
        p.   cm.
    Sinskey's name appears first on previous ed.
    Includes bibliographical references and index.
    ISBN 0-7506-7082-7
    1. Cataract--Surgery Handbooks, manuals, etc. I. Sinskey, Robert
M. II. Title.
    [DNLM: 1. Cataract Extraction--methods Handbooks. WW 39 B151m
2000]
RE451.S56 2000
617.7'42059--dc21
DNLM/DLC
for Library of Congress   99-29627
                                                             CIP

British Library Cataloguing-in-Publication Data
A catalogue record for this book is available from the British Library.

The publisher offers special discounts on bulk orders of this book.
For information, please contact:

Manager of Special Sales
Butterworth–Heinemann
225 Wildwood Avenue
Woburn, MA 01801-2041
Tel: 781-904-2500
Fax: 781-904-2620

For information on all Butterworth–Heinemann publications available,
contact our World Wide Web home page at: http://www.bh.com

10 9 8 7 6 5 4 3 2 1

Printed in the United States of America

Contents

Author Biographies

Gavin G. Bahadur, M.D.
Cataract and Anterior Segment Surgeon, The Sinskey Eye Institute, Santa Monica, California; Active Staff, Department of Ophthalmology, St. John's Hospital and Medical Center, Santa Monica

Gavin G. Bahadur, M.D., is an anterior segment surgeon at The Sinskey Eye Institute. Dr. Bahadur completed his residency and fellowship at the Manhattan Eye, Ear & Throat Hospital in New York, where he conducted focused training in cataract, cornea, glaucoma, and refractive surgery and served as a clinical instructor. Dr. Bahadur assisted in the development of the latest cataract techniques, including research on neodymium:yttrium-aluminum garnet laser phacolysis. He has instructed physicians in training, instructed eye surgeons on a variety of ophthalmic surgical procedures, and written textbook chapters on advanced techniques in cataract surgery. Dr. Bahadur has made presentations at the American Academy of Ophthalmology, the Association for Research in Vision and Ophthalmology, and the International Society of Refractive Surgery and has conducted scientific research at the National Institutes of Health, the Brown University School of Medicine, and the Duke University Eye Center.

Robert M. Sinskey, M.D.
Clinical Professor of Ophthalmology, Jules Stein Eye Institute, University of California, Los Angeles, UCLA School of Medicine; Active Staff, Department of Ophthalmology, St. John's Hospital and Medical Center, Santa Monica, California

Robert M. Sinskey, M.D., the founder of The Sinskey Eye Institute in Santa Monica, California, is also Clinical Professor of Ophthalmology at the Jules Stein Eye Institute, University of California, Los Angeles; President of the American Society of Cataract and Refractive Surgery, 1999–2000; President of the Foundation for Ophthalmic Education; and a member of the medical staff at St. John's Hospital and Santa Monica Hospital. He is on the editorial boards of *Ocular Surgery News*, *Ophthalmology Times*, *European Journal of Implant and Refractive Surgery*, and *Asia Pacific Journal of Ophthalmology*. Dr. Sinskey has been a guest faculty member and surgeon in more than 100 symposia all over the world; has had more than 200 speaking engagements in the United States, North America, South America, Asia, Europe and Africa; and has had more than 30 journal publications. Dr. Sinskey patented the

Sinskey Modified "J" Loop Intraocular Lens, one of the most popular intraocular lens implants in the world and has invented a number of surgical techniques and instruments, notably the ubiquitous Sinskey hook. Dr. Sinskey pioneered posterior chamber phacoemulsification, the use of low-power intraocular lens implants, and intraocular lens implants in infants and children.

Foreword

This manual represents the collaborative effort of an extremely well-trained young surgeon, Gavin G. Bahadur, M.D., and one of the most experienced and respected cataract surgeons in the world, Robert M. Sinskey, M.D. The rapid change in cataract surgery technology and technique is still supported by certain underlying principles. This manual reviews those principles without being too technical or mired in minutiae. Although there will not be universal agreement with all of the preferences of the authors, the comprehensive approach to cataract surgery presented here is an appropriate point of embarkation for surgeons in training. The step-by-step approach, adequately documented with literature references and illustrated with diagrams, facilitates learning for those in training and affords rapid review for more senior surgeons. This concise and easy-to-read manual is a beneficial resource for all ophthalmologists interested in cataract surgery.

Dr. Sinskey has contributed to training the majority of surgeons practicing phacoemulsification today. This manual extends that contribution and passes the torch to a new generation of anterior segment surgeons.

I. Howard Fine

Preface

We have written this book for ophthalmology residents and fellows and for surgeons who want to refine their techniques or add to their surgical armamentarium. Some of the techniques outlined here are the authors' favored routine methods, whereas others are mentioned for their advantages in particular situations. We recognize that there are multiple methods for achieving a successful result, and part of our goal is to identify the advantages and pitfalls of a variety of approaches.

A mere text is no substitute for years of experience and self-criticism. The reader is encouraged to continually refine techniques with good observation and the use of surgical videotapes. We hope that our text will provide a logical foundation for the treatment of your patients.

G.G.B.
R.M.S.

Note: The authors have no financial interests in any ophthalmologic devices or products discussed in this book.

Acknowledgments

Very special thanks to Dr. Jay Patel for all his work on the original edition of this text 12 years ago.

We are indebted to our illustrator, Laurel Cook Lhowe, for her ability to transform mere words into detailed yet clear drawings and for her patience with subtle revisions.

We would also like to acknowledge the efforts of Jayne Gordon for her tireless assistance in typing the manuscript. Thanks also to Leslie Kramer and Karen Oberheim at Butterworth–Heinemann, Dr. Harvey Gutman, Dr. Lawrence Garwood, and Dr. Jerry Pierce for their support and assistance.

G.G.B.
R.M.S.

Manual of Cataract Surgery

Chapter 1
Preoperative Evaluation

The preoperative evaluation of a potential cataract surgery patient includes a complete ocular and medical history and a comprehensive ophthalmologic examination. The most significant decision a surgeon makes is whether to operate in the first place. An honest and detailed discussion with the patient during the examination is essential to ensure that the patient's expectations of surgery are realistic and warranted.

Remember that the risks of surgery are relative. In a patient with bare–light-perception vision, the remote risk of loss of the eye secondary to endophthalmitis may be almost inconsequential. In a patient with mild nocturnal glare symptoms, the risk of chronic cystoid macular edema (CME) may be cause for concern. The patient and surgeon must share the responsibility of accepting the risks of the planned procedure.

Before surgery is scheduled, the following questions should be answered to the satisfaction of the physician and patient:

1. Is the patient expected to benefit from the operation?
2. Is the patient willing to accept the risks of surgery?
3. Is the surgery necessary, given the patient's lifestyle?

It is not our intent here to discuss in detail the critical arts of examination and history taking, but instead to emphasize the key points that help to answer these questions.

Ocular History

The purpose of the ocular history is to

1. Assess how the patient's activities and quality of life are affected by visual limitations. Determine if perceived visual deficits exist that impact the patient's daily activities, occupation, hobbies, or future plans.
2. Establish whether the patient's visual symptoms are consistent with the presence of cataracts. Ask about visual clarity, glare, and the brightness of colors. If visual acuity fluctuates even in unchanging lighting conditions, then cataracts are an unlikely source of the patient's symptoms.
3. Identify concomitant conditions, such as pseudo-exfoliation, lens subluxation or dislocation, zonular dehiscence, glaucoma, high myopia, retinal breaks, retinal detachments, macular holes or cysts, macular degeneration, vascular diseases (including diabetes and hypertension), trauma, or cerebrovascular accidents.
4. Evaluate the outcome of cataract surgery in the fellow eye, if applicable. Identify potential causes of, or risk factors for, complications in the fellow eye, such as poor dilatation, weak zonules, a bleeding diathesis, a dense nucleus, or corneal disease.
5. Evaluate the patient's perception of his or her visual acuity before the development of the cataract. Was there a time when the patient noted clearer vision in the cataractous eye? If the patient has

never had better vision in the affected eye, possibilities such as amblyopia, retinal disease, or optic neuropathy should be explored. Although there may be a significant cataract in the presence of these diagnoses, cataract surgery may be of little or no benefit to the patient. Above all, the surgeon should never subject a patient to an operation that is of no perceived visual benefit.

6. Establish the patient's expectations of cataract surgery. Determine the patient's need for distant versus near vision. Determine whether the patient would prefer to be emmetropic or slightly myopic after the surgery. Is the patient a candidate for monovision or a multifocal lens? Take into consideration the patient's occupation, hobbies, interests and desires; every patient has a unique personality and individualized visual needs.

Medical History

The general medical status of the patient should be evaluated before performing surgery. Consulting with the patient's internist and the anesthesiologist will determine whether the patient is in sound medical condition. It may be helpful to inform the internist of the relatively low systemic risks of cataract surgery and that surgery is an option even if the patient is anticoagulated. Once the patient is cleared for surgery by the internist, the surgeon and anesthesiologist should become familiar with any medical conditions that could affect the surgical outcome or influence their judgment in the event of a medical emergency unrelated to the surgery.

Cardiac Disease

During surgery, patients with potentially compromised coronary blood flow should be monitored closely for symptoms of angina or changes in vital signs. When appropriate, medical clearance should be obtained from the patient's cardiologist before scheduling the procedure. The surgeon should be prepared to pause or even terminate the procedure in the event of an attack of angina or an acute myocardial infarction. These possibilities should be discussed with the patient during the informed-consent process. The use of self-sealing incisions or

preplaced sutures clearly facilitates rapid wound closure in such emergency situations.

Airway

Patients with emphysema, chronic bronchitis, asthma, congestive heart failure, or other respiratory conditions require special attention during surgery. The patient's body position should maximize airway patency and the comfort of patient and surgeon. If it is impossible to optimize all of these factors simultaneously, the surgeon and anesthesiologist should determine the best compromise. Tenting the surgical drape a few inches above the patient's mouth and nose by draping it over the Mayo instrument stand minimizes the claustrophobic effect on the patient. Additionally, a two-pronged nasal cannula or flexible oxygen tubing attached to 2–5 liters of oxygen per minute is helpful to ensure an adequate oxygen supply.

Dentures, if present, should be assessed for fit before surgery. Well-fitting dentures help to open the airway, while loose dentures may be displaced during surgery and block the airway. The anesthesiologist should support the jaw to ensure a patent airway.

Congestive Heart Failure

Patients with compromised venous return may have congested episcleral veins, which can elevate intraocular pressure (IOP). It may be tempting to consider an osmotic diuretic to dehydrate the vitreous before surgery; however, hyperosmotic agents can vastly increase intravascular volume and are generally contraindicated in congestive heart failure. In patients with orthopnea, the head and chest should be elevated to a position that still allows comfortable access to the globe.

Hypertension and Atherosclerosis

Hypertension and atherosclerotic disease are risk factors for expulsive suprachoroidal hemorrhage, retrobulbar hemorrhage, and conjunctival and iris bleeding. These possibilities should be discussed with the patient during the informed-consent process, and the surgeon should adjust the approach accordingly. Using topical anesthesia in such cases lowers the probability of a retrobulbar hemorrhage secondary to intraorbital injection. An appropriately sized, clear, self-sealing corneal incision helps the surgeon avoid conjunctival vessels and promotes a tight seal during phacoemulsification, decreasing the likelihood of a suprachoroidal hemorrhage.

Diabetes Mellitus

A cataract patient with diabetes often poses an interesting management challenge. Removal of the cataractous lens and replacement with an intraocular lens (IOL) implant improves the patient's vision and facilitates examination and possible treatment of diabetic retinopathy. On the other hand, the inflammatory mediators liberated by cataract surgery itself have been implicated in the acceleration of diabetic retinal changes, including the exacerbation of clinically significant macular edema.

Even if a patient is only mildly visually symptomatic, cataract extraction with IOL should be considered if (1) a dense cataract prevents adequate examination of the retina, (2) lenticular opacity blocks transmission of laser energy when panretinal photocoagulation is performed, or (3) the cataract prevents the surgical visualization necessary for vitrectomy surgery.

Careful preoperative fundoscopic evaluation is necessary to evaluate diabetic retinopathy. The possibility of exacerbating clinically significant macular edema should be considered and discussed with the patient. The anesthesiologist may wish to consult with the patient's internist or endocrinologist to determine the optimal dose of insulin or oral hypoglycemic agent during the nothing-by-mouth (NPO) period before surgery. Consideration should be given to scheduling diabetic patients early in the morning to minimize their waking hours without oral intake. Increased susceptibility to infection and the possibility of impaired wound healing should be kept in mind during the postoperative follow-up.

Musculoskeletal Disorders

Patients with severe spinal disorders, such as kyphosis or scoliosis, may be difficult to position on the operating table. A specially designed operating table that can be flexed or laterally tilted may alleviate this problem. It is essential for the operating table to include an articulating headrest that can be positioned independently of the table proper. Patients with rheumatoid arthritis may have severe disease involving the odontoid process, which can pose a significant intubation risk in cases with general anesthesia.

Alcoholism, Recreational Drug Use, and Chronic Pain

Patients with alcoholism, a history of recreational drug use, and chronic pain may require higher-than-average doses of anesthetics caused by up-regulation of metabolism and down-regulation of receptors. The surgeon should be particularly watchful for signs of pain, withdrawal, agitation, or confusion.

Tobacco Use

Tobacco smoking can decrease the oxygen-carrying capacity of blood owing to the binding of carbon monoxide to hemoglobin. Care should be taken to ensure that smokers have an adequate oxygen supply throughout the procedure. A nasal cannula or unobtrusive oxygen mask may be used. Additionally, the surgeon should be aware that smokers may be more likely to cough during the procedure. It is helpful to ask the patient to warn the surgeon, whenever possible, of an impending cough.

Steroids

Patients with asthma, arthritis, connective-tissue disorders, or other conditions requiring chronic steroid use may exhibit delayed wound healing or an increased incidence of bleeding complications. Due to suppression of the adrenal axis, these patients may require higher-than-usual postoperative doses of steroids for effective modulation of the inflammatory response. The patient should be warned of the possible risks of glaucoma and cataracts secondary to steroid use.

Bleeding Disorders

Iatrogenic anticoagulation with aspirin- or warfarin-containing compounds is the most common form of bleeding diathesis encountered. The surgeon should be mindful of conditions, such as hemophilia or thrombocytopenia, that can alter clotting times. If medically appropriate, the surgeon may wish to work with an internist or hematologist to normalize clotting parameters before surgery. If this is not possible, or is medically contraindicated, then a detailed discussion with the patient is necessary to outline the risks of retrobulbar hemorrhage, choroidal hemorrhage, hyphema, and subconjunctival hemorrhage. Topical anesthesia with clear corneal incisions should be considered in these cases. If an anterior chamber (AC) lens is placed, consider performing a laser iridotomy postoperatively, in place of a surgical iridectomy to reduce the risk of hyphema.

Medications

A survey of the patient's systemic medications, especially those affecting coagulation parameters, is essential. Warfarin, acetylsalicylic acid, and nonsteroidal anti-inflammatory drugs (NSAIDs) can affect clotting time. The patient's internist must be consulted before stopping any anticoagulants. If holding anticoagulant therapy is contraindicated, clear corneal phacoemulsification with topical anesthesia should be considered, and the risks and benefits should be discussed in detail with the patient, as described above. Patients on antihypertensive medications may have a contracted vascular compartment; if considering the administration of intravenous solutions such as mannitol, serum electrolytes should be monitored.

Ocular medications, such as phospholine iodide and pilocarpine, can result in small, poorly reactive pupils. Prostaglandin analogs, such as latanoprost, can exacerbate CME.

Ophthalmic Examination

A thorough preoperative examination, including the components listed in the following sections, is essential.

External Examination

Any open skin lesions or rashes in the periorbital area should be addressed and treated before surgery.

Acyclovir prophylaxis should be considered in patients with a history of herpes zoster affecting the ophthalmic division of the trigeminal nerve. Prominent brows or deeply sunken orbits should be noted, as these features may affect operative positioning.

Extraocular Movements

Any tropias or significant phorias should be measured and noted. The risk of binocular diplopia and the possible need for subsequent prism correction or strabismus surgery should be discussed with the patient to establish realistic goals, and appropriate informed consent should be obtained.

Visual Acuity

Although specific visual acuity parameters may be necessary for some insurance carriers, it is the functional acuity that is of greatest concern to the patient. The American Academy of Ophthalmology and the Health Care Financing Administration (under the U.S. Department of Health and Human Services) each have their own guidelines for visual assessment that may influence your evaluation. Brightness acuity testing may be useful to quantitate glare disability, and some third-party payers may require its documentation.

Because each patient is unique, a universal visual-acuity threshold is not an appropriate guide for planning cataract surgery. For example, a patient whose favorite pastime is listening to symphony recordings may not experience the same visual symptoms as an airplane pilot. A detailed history and discussion of the patient's visual needs are essential for appropriate patient selection.

Pupils

The presence of an afferent pupillary defect indicates optic nerve pathology or severe retinal compromise and generally heralds a poor prognosis for visual potential after cataract surgery. Irregular or small pupils in the presence of dilating medications should be noted, as these findings may influence surgical technique.

Lids, Lashes, and Lacrimal Apparatus

Any infectious or inflammatory diseases of the eyelids, lashes, or ocular adnexa (such as blepharitis or dacryocystitis) should be treated before surgery to reduce the risk of endophthalmitis. Low-grade, chronic, staphylococcal blepharitis, for example, should be managed with a combination of warm compresses, eyelid and lash hygiene, and topical eyedrops or ophthalmic ointments. The use of routine preoperative antibiotics in the absence of lid disease does not appear to be of significant clinical benefit.

A dry-eye condition should be identified and treated, as this may affect postoperative patient comfort and wound healing. Entropion, ectropion, or lid laxity should be addressed before surgery, as these abnormalities can disrupt tear-film integrity and impair healing of the ocular surface.

Any ptosis or asymmetry in the palpebral fissures should be noted. Depending on operative technique, cataract surgery can exacerbate levator dehiscence in some cases.

Conjunctiva and Sclera

The presence of a pterygium or significant pingueculum should be noted and addressed, as these may induce astigmatic changes and can influence the location of the cataract incision. In some cases, it may be prudent to excise a pterygium at the time of cataract extraction.

Cornea

The presence of corneal lesions or active corneal pathology is important to identify preoperatively. Central corneal opacities may obscure the surgeon's view intraoperatively, making some steps quite challenging. Severe pannus may influence the incision location and may also affect astigmatic results. The presence of significant guttata or mild corneal edema influences the discussion of risks and benefits of the surgery, and a penetrating keratoplasty may be required after the cataract surgery. Remember that quick, atraumatic cataract surgery may have little effect on endothelial status. In cases of severe preoperative corneal opacification, consideration should be given to a combined procedure that includes a penetrating keratoplasty.

Anterior Chamber

AC depth and the presence of any inflammation are important in the preoperative evaluation. The shallow AC of a hyperopic eye can complicate wound construction, the stability of chamber depth, and wound closure. Conversely, the large AC of a myopic eye can result in large amplitude shifts in the position of the posterior capsule as instruments are introduced and removed from the eye during surgery.

Ideally, the patient should be free of uveitis for at least 4 months before surgery, although this may not always be possible. In some cases, prophylactic acyclovir may be indicated to reduce the likelihood of postoperative herpetic recurrences.

Iris

Anterior or posterior synechiae should be noted, as these can complicate surgery. Posterior synechiae are usually lysed at the start of the procedure to facilitate pupillary dilation. Peripheral anterior synechiae can result in elevated IOP postoperatively. With practice and care, cataract surgery can be performed successfully with little or no manipulation of the iris.

Lens

Although some correlation exists between the slit-lamp appearance of a lens and the actual density of the nucleus, even the most experienced cataract surgeons are often surprised by intraoperative lenticular consistency. Nonetheless, the lens should be carefully examined, with particular attention given to the degree of nuclear sclerosis, posterior subcapsular (PSC) opacity, polar opacity, hypermaturity of the lens, phacodonesis, subluxation or decentration, and capsular disruption. It is important to note the quality of the red reflex, as this can have tremendous impact on the ease of creating a capsulorhexis and of subsequent phacoemulsification. The red reflex may be affected by cortical spokes, lamellar opacities, cloudy hypermature lens, dense brunescent nuclear sclerosis, or by posterior segment findings such as dense asteroid hyalosis, vitreous hemorrhage, or retinal detachment.

Intraocular Pressure

Signs of glaucoma, including IOP, should be evaluated and treated if necessary before cataract surgery. If glaucomatous progression occurs in the setting of a visually significant cataract, combined cataract extraction with trabeculectomy should be considered, as cataract surgery alone may have an IOP-lowering effect (Tennen 1996; Murchison 1989). Our understanding of glaucoma mechanisms is evolving rapidly, and controversy exists regarding the indications for combined trabeculectomy and cataract and implant surgery.

In patients with significant visual field loss or glaucomatous optic nerve cupping, IOP-lowering agents should be used at the conclusion of surgery to guard against postoperative IOP spikes. In patients with profound glaucomatous optic nerve damage, cataract surgery should be performed in the morning, and IOP should be checked that afternoon and the following morning. In this setting, even a transient IOP spike may critically damage the remaining optic nerve fibers.

It is important to recognize the signs of phacomorphic glaucoma: elevated IOP in the setting of significant nuclear sclerosis, shallowing of the AC, and narrowing of the angle. In many of these cases, removal of the cataract alone causes a dramatic widening of the angle and a lowering of IOP.

Optic Neuropathies

The presence of significant cupping or pallor secondary to glaucoma, anterior ischemic optic neuropathy, optic neuritis, or other conditions may reduce postoperative visual potential and should be discussed with the patient to ensure realistic expectations. Furthermore, significant optic nerve damage may be aggravated by perioperative elevations in pressure, as may occur with the use of a Honan balloon, excessive infusion through a tight wound, or postoperative IOP spikes.

Vitreous and Retina

Examination of the vitreous and retina is essential for predicting postoperative visual potential and for identifying risk factors for CME or retinal detachment. Retinal holes, tears, or detachments should be treated before cataract surgery, and underlying retinal disease, such as diabetic retinopathy or macular degeneration, should be addressed. The presence of nonclearing vitreous hemorrhage may necessitate a combined vitrectomy. Asteroid hyalosis, although benign, can prove quite distracting to the surgeon and may adversely affect postoperative vision.

If the cataract causes a media opacity that obscures the view of the vitreous or retina, a potential acuity meter, B-scan ultrasound, bright-flash electroretinogram (ERG), or entoptic phenomena should be used singly or in combination to assist in predicting visual potential.

Ancillary Ophthalmic Testing

Intraocular Lens Power Determination

A-Scan Ultrasonography

An accurate axial-length measurement (A-scan) is required if the patient is scheduled for IOL implantation. The same operator should perform all A-scans to eliminate interobserver variation and to achieve consistent, reproducible results. Multiple axial-length measurements should be taken until reproducibility is achieved. Care should be taken to avoid distortion of the globe during measurements. An immersion A-scan may help to maximize reproducibility, but is not well-tolerated by all patients. Measurement of the fellow eye is often extremely useful for purposes of comparison, with the understanding that variations in axial length between the two eyes do occur.

Corneal Curvature

Accurate keratometry to determine corneal refractive power is required for IOL power calculation. As with A-scan measurements, consistency is crucial and interobserver variation should be minimized whenever possible. Measurements by one observer should be repeated at least three times or until consistent readings are obtained.

Corneal topography is an extremely useful adjunct to keratometry and can help confirm keratometric readings. In addition, topography is indispensable when planning incision location. The incision can be placed in the steepest topographic meridian, allowing the relaxing effect of the wound to minimize astigmatic effects and reduce or eliminate a pre-existing cylinder.

In the future, an increasing number of patients will have cataract surgery after undergoing refractive surgery (e.g., radial keratotomy, photorefractive keratectomy, laser-assisted in situ keratomileusis, and intrastromal corneal ring segments). Corneal topography in conjunction with empiric nomograms is extremely valuable in assessing the effects of corneal curvature on IOL power calculations.

Intraocular Lens Power Calculation

Numerous IOL calculation programs are available. Regardless of the program used, taking into account factors unique to the surgeon and A-scan technician is essential to achieve accurate results. Cases should be periodically reviewed to compare actual postoperative refractions with predicted values, and adjustments to IOL power selection should be made accordingly. Standardizing incision architecture and other surgical techniques promote consistent results. Always remember to compensate for any changes in the A-constant when using a different IOL model.

Once personalized factors are taken into account, a variety of IOL power formulas may be used, including SRK II, SRK/T, Holladay, and Hoffer Q (Flowers et al. 1996). If prior cataract surgery has been performed on the fellow eye with an IOL, use the difference between the actual and predicted refractive results to help guide your choice of lens power in the current operative eye.

If an IOL must be placed in the ciliary sulcus rather than in the capsular bag, remember to compensate by decreasing IOL power. Although the adjustment is usually 0.50 to 0.75 diopters, the most accurate way to determine the magnitude of the IOL power adjustment is to review your own cases.

Tests of Visual Potential

Fixation on a Light

A very simple test of macular function in a patient with a dense cataract is fixation on a point source of light. Ask the patient to fix and follow a bright muscle light, and observe whether the patient follows smoothly, without random, searching eye movements. Although some cataracts can scatter light sources to a diffuse blur, patients with healthy macular function may still be able to pinpoint and accurately follow the light source. Although this test is by no means quantitative, it is simple and yields a quick prediction of visual potential.

Potential Acuity Meter

Developed by Guyton and Minkowski (Minkowski 1983), the potential acuity meter (PAM) projects a Snellen's chart onto the retina through the small clear optical zone within a cataract or other media opacity. The test can be useful for predicting postoperative acuity, but like many tests of macular function, its accuracy is limited.

Vitreous opacities, extremely dense nuclei, PSC cataracts, and testing through a miotic pupil can all lead to an underestimation of true potential acuity. A scanning laser ophthalmoscope may be particularly useful in cases with PSC cataracts in which the long-wavelength HeNe laser beam is less scattered by the opacity than the white light of the PAM (Cuzzani et al. 1998). Disorders resulting in an overestimation of postoperative visual acuity include cystoid macular edema, macular holes with cysts, epiretinal membranes, central serous chorioretinopathy, and early shallow retinal detachments. Age-related macular degeneration may result in false-positives or false-negatives.

Interferometers

The interferometer measures interference patterns produced by coherent light sources. The patient is asked to identify the orientation of these interference fringes as they are projected through a dilatated pupil. The instrument allows the operator to alter the width of the interference bands and correlate them with various potential visual acuities.

Entoptic Phenomena

The "Flying Corpuscle." In the "flying corpuscle" test, the patient views a uniform blue screen. The blue light is absorbed by the retinal capillaries, preventing it from reaching the photoreceptors, while white blood cells traversing the capillaries allow the light to be transmitted, stimulating the photoreceptors and resulting in the image of a particle moving across the visual field. The predicted visual acuity is thought to be at least 20/200. This test is of limited value in patients with severe opacities (which prevent the blue light from reaching the retinal vessels) and in patients unable to appreciate the effect.

Purkinje's Vascular Entoptic Test. Purkinje's vascular entoptic test is a second method used to elicit an entoptic response that involves placing a bright transilluminator against the closed eyelid and moving it back and forth, creating images of the patient's vascular tree. Patients who can identify the foveal avascular zone are predicted to have visual acuities of 20/40 or greater. Like all entoptic measures, Purkinje's test is limited by the patient's subjective interpretations.

B-Scan Ultrasonography

In the case of a lens opacity that is too dense for biomicroscopy of the fundus, a B-scan ultrasound should be performed to rule out retinal detachment, vitreous hemorrhage, tumors, and other posterior segment pathology. A retina consultation and appropriate workup should be obtained before scheduling cataract surgery, if indicated by the B-scan findings.

Specular Microscopy

Endothelial cell count and evaluation of the endothelial cell mosaic with specular microscopy are rarely indicated in our current management of cataracts, except possibly in the case of:

1. Unexplained corneal decompensation after uneventful cataract surgery in the fellow eye.
2. Signs of significant Descemet's membrane or endothelial compromise.
3. Research on the effects of new surgical techniques and intraoperative medications.

If an endothelial cell count is obtained, it is imperative to remember that endothelial cell density does not necessarily correlate with endothelial cell function or ultimate visual potential. Corneas with endothelial cell counts of 600 cells/mm^2 may remain clear after cataract surgery, while those with more than 2,000 cells/mm^2 may not. Nonetheless, in patients at risk for corneal decompensation, specular microscopy may be a helpful component of medicolegal documentation and may influence the discussion of the relative risks and benefits of the proposed procedure. The advent of noncontact specular microscopy makes the testing much simpler for the patient.

Preoperative Medical Clearance

The requirements for preoperative testing vary widely among hospitals and surgery centers. Although an uncomplicated, clear corneal phacoemulsification under topical anesthesia may seem no more traumatic than a minor room procedure, the potential for unforeseen complications certainly exists. The surgeon and anesthesiologist should work in concert to determine the most appropriate and reasonable workup for preoperative medical clearance. Ideally, medical clearance should be obtained with the help of the patient's primary care physician. Patients at high risk for stroke, myocardial infarction, angina, dyspnea, wheezing, labile hypertension, or diabetes may require specialist consultation. As a guideline, the following tests should be considered: an electrolyte panel; a complete blood cell count, including platelets; a chest x-ray; and an electrocardiogram.

Chapter 2
Anesthesia

The purpose of anesthesia is to safely provide comfort for the patient while optimizing conditions for the surgeon. Cataract surgeons have a variety of anesthesia options.

The Anesthesiologist

The primary goal of an elective procedure is patient safety. Having a qualified anesthesiologist in the operating room is essential for the prompt management of medical emergencies.

In the hands of a skilled surgeon, cataract surgery is a routine procedure requiring no more than a few minutes. Although it may be tempting to operate without an anesthesiologist, the surgeon should never forget the demographic cataract patients are typically drawn from. Such patients tend to be elderly, with concomitant medical conditions such as cardiovascular disease, hypertension, and diabetes. Although the need for an anesthesiologist during a brief, uncomplicated phacoemulsification under topical anesthesia is debated, an anesthesiologist is clearly indispensable in an ostensibly routine case in which complications, such as vitreous loss, iris prolapse, or corneal clouding, occur and the patient becomes acutely hypertensive, agitated, or dyspneic. Although these examples may seem extreme, such situations are likely to arise in a busy practice.

The potential for life-threatening complications during any surgery cannot be ignored. When a medical emergency suddenly arises during an already difficult procedure, an anesthesiologist is invaluable for the well-being of both the patient and the surgeon.

Selection of Anesthesia

A number of factors influence the choice of anesthesia, including

1. The anticipated complexity and duration of the surgical procedure.
2. The patient's medical status (e.g., the presence of cardiopulmonary disease or coagulopathy).
3. The patient's emotional status and ability to cooperate.
4. The surgeon's skill and preference.
5. The anesthesiologist's skill and preference.

Every patient is different. Recognizing the specific needs and desires of each patient permits you to select the anesthesia, surgical technique, and IOL most appropriate for each case.

Anesthesiologist's Evaluation

The anesthesiologist's preoperative evaluation of the patient is critical for selecting the appropriate anesthetic approach. During this visit, the anesthesiologist establishes a rapport with the patient and attempts to relieve anxiety; this can even reduce or eliminate the need for preoperative sedation. The anesthesiologist reviews the pertinent medical history, which may affect the selection of anesthetic agents. The goal is to have a calm, relaxed, cooperative patient in the operating room.

Nothing-by-Mouth Instructions

The risk of airway compromise resulting from aspiration in patients under NPO instructions has decreased significantly with the advent of topical and intracameral anesthetic techniques. Often, cataract surgery patients require no intravenous sedation and maintain excellent airway control. Nonetheless, the remote but potentially catastrophic risk of aspiration should be addressed, especially in patients with a history of gastroesophageal reflux disease.

When cases are scheduled for late in the day, strict NPO instructions after midnight the night before surgery may result in light-headedness, headache, nausea, or blood pressure elevation. For these patients, it is best to allow a light diet consisting of clear fluids and jam and toast on the morning of surgery, provided general anesthesia is not planned. High-protein-content foods should be avoided, as these can delay gastric emptying. If necessary, metoclopramide may be used to promote peristalsis and prevent nausea.

Anesthetic Agents

Propofol

Propofol is a sedative-hypnotic with an extremely rapid onset of action. It allows a quick recovery to a lucid state with little postoperative nausea and vomiting. The anesthesiologist must be watchful for hypotension secondary to vasodilation and cardiac depression. Propofol can cause a dose-dependent decrease in cerebral perfusion, resulting in apnea. However, the medication may also have the desirable effect of lowering IOP (White 1997). The injection of propofol into small-caliber veins is commonly painful; injecting lidocaine before injecting the propofol may significantly reduce discomfort (Wetchler 1991).

Narcotics

Narcotics facilitate the induction of general anesthesia. They have effective analgesic properties, prevent coughing, and often lower IOP. Nausea and vomiting are common side effects.

Fentanyl is a synthetic narcotic with an extremely rapid onset of action. It can reduce the discomfort associated with local blocks in the conscious patient (Wetchler 1991).

Sedatives

Sedatives of the phenothiazine class were once frequently used as an anesthetic for their sedative, antiarrhythmic, and antiemetic effects. However, these medications have a long duration of action, may induce dizziness, and can cause hypotension. Far better alternatives are now available.

Benzodiazepines

Diazepam

Diazepam, one of the most commonly used sedatives, can be administered orally or intravenously and has excellent anxiolytic, sedative, and amnestic properties. Patients should be monitored for respiratory and cardiovascular depression (Wetchler 1991). Oral diazepam can relieve anxiety, cause mild sedation, and promote comfort. The injection of intravenous diazepam can be painful, and its duration of action may be undesirably long. The depth of sedation is critical during a case; oversedation with diazepam can cause confusion and counterproductive movements resulting from snoring, particularly in geriatric patients.

Midazolam

Midazolam is a popular and effective intravenous medication used to achieve sedation, reduce anxiety, create anterograde amnesia, and, in carefully titrated doses, enhance cooperation. Midazolam has a rapid onset of action, and, unlike diazepam, its injection causes little discomfort. Midazolam can result in dose-related respiratory depression, and its amnestic effects must be kept in mind when explaining postoperative instructions to the patient. It is helpful to have a friend or family member present postoperatively to help with any discharge instructions (White 1997). Keep in mind that benzodiazepines have no analgesic properties, and may even cause paradoxical restlessness when administered to patients experiencing pain (Wetchler 1991).

Anticholinergics

Anticholinergic medications are rarely used in cataract surgery, but may be useful for decreasing upper respiratory tract secretions and preventing the oculocardiac reflex. Dry mouth is a common side effect. Intramuscular atropine and glycopyrrolate are common choices. In general, scopolamine should be avoided, as it can cause restlessness and disorientation in elderly patients.

Local Anesthetic Techniques

Regional blocks are quite popular in cataract surgery because of their relative safety and reliability in producing anesthesia and akinesia. Before the administration of a regional nerve block, a sedating agent is recommended for anxiolysis and for maximizing patient cooperation and comfort. Pre-emptive anesthesia to prevent pain also helps reduce nausea and anxiety; administering anesthetic agents after the onset of pain results in discomfort and anxiety.

The anesthesiologist should be prepared for the respiratory depression that can result from the administration of a sedative. The airway should be kept open at all times. Coughing, sneezing, or laryngospasm may also occur.

Local Anesthetic Agents

For a retrobulbar or peribulbar block, a 50:50 compounded solution of 0.4% lidocaine with 0.75% bupivacaine is an excellent mixture for producing akinesia and anesthesia. Lidocaine has a rapid onset of action, while bupivacaine has a

longer duration. Depending on the time interval between the administration of the block and the start of surgery, 0.75% bupivacaine alone may be used; its onset of action is 10 minutes or less. The use of lidocaine alone may be helpful in a monocular patient requiring rapid postoperative visual rehabilitation.

The addition of 150 units of hyaluronidase causes rapid diffusion of the anesthetic agent, thereby accelerating the onset of action of a regional block (Mindel 1978). Hyaluronidase should be used with caution, as it may cause anesthesia in nontarget tissues. Hyaluronidase should not be used, for example, with Nadbath or O'Brien blocks because of the risk of anesthesia infiltrating the adjacent muscles of mastication and swallowing. Hyaluronidase may be used in Van Lint or Atkinson blocks.

Vasoconstrictors may be useful for facial nerve blocks to prolong their duration, but should not be used with long-acting anesthetic agents.

Retrobulbar Anesthesia

Akinesia of the globe is clearly advantageous during intraocular surgery, especially for the inexperienced surgeon. The time-honored technique for achieving globe akinesia is the injection of local anesthetic into the muscle cone in the retrobulbar space. An effective retrobulbar block results in ocular akinesia, anesthesia of the ocular surface, and internal ophthalmoplegia of the iris sphincter and ciliary muscle. The choice of the anesthetic agent is left to the surgeon. The surgeon should be familiar with the duration of action, side effects, and toxic effects of the anesthetic(s) chosen.

Retrobulbar Block Technique

The following steps describe the induction of anesthesia using a retrobulbar block technique:

1. Use a sharp or dull 1.5-in., 25-gauge needle with a 5-ml syringe. A dull Atkinson needle is less likely to damage a nerve or vessel and offers better tactile cues about the intramuscular septum as the muscle cone is entered; on the other hand, a sharp needle enters the skin more easily and may cause

less trauma than a dull needle in the event of globe penetration (White 1997).

2. Administer an appropriate amount of intravenous sedation to the patient.

3. Instill topical proparacaine in the upper and lower conjunctival fornices. Tetracaine may be used as an alternative, but is more toxic to the corneal epithelium. The topical anesthetic serves two purposes: The patient's blink reflex is attenuated, and the cornea is anesthetized before the alcohol swab used in skin preparation is applied.

4. Palpate the inferior orbital margin at its outer one-third. Cleanse the skin in this area with an alcohol swab.

5. If minimal sedation is used, direct the patient to gaze slightly inferotemporally or in primary gaze, which keeps the optic nerve out of the needle's path.

6. Introduce the needle along the inferior orbital rim at the junction of its outer one-third and inner two-thirds. The needle should be parallel to the orbital floor for approximately the first 1 cm of its insertion, then directed medially toward the orbital apex as it is advanced posteriorly. As the muscle cone is entered, resistance can frequently be felt if the Atkinson needle is used. Never advance the needle to its hub, instead leaving approximately 0.5 cm visible above the skin.

7. Aspirate with the plunger. If blood is visible in the syringe, discontinue the procedure and withdraw the needle to avoid intravascular or intrathecal injection of anesthetic. Use a peribulbar block as an alternative or defer the surgery.

8. If no blood is seen in the syringe, perform a slow deliberate injection of the anesthetic agent with infiltration along the track of the needle as it is withdrawn (Gills and Loyd 1983). If the retrobulbar injection is given after the patient is rendered unconscious using a short-acting barbiturate, the same steps are followed, except that the surgeon is unable to ask the patient to direct his or her gaze. Nevertheless, excellent retrobulbar anesthesia can be achieved.

9. Immediately after withdrawing the needle, close the lids and apply pressure to the eye with the flat of the hand over a gauze square. Maintain pressure for approximately 60 seconds. If considerable proptosis exists or the globe feels firm, apply additional pressure, but for no longer than 60 seconds at a time. Retract the lids manually and examine the eye for signs of retrobulbar hemorrhage. Assess the adequacy of the block by directing the patient to gaze in various directions. Although some degree of superior oblique action is often present, this is of little or no consequence. If a short-acting barbiturate was used, the surgeon and anesthesiologist must ensure that the patient is returning to consciousness and breathing spontaneously. Support the lower jaw with your fingers under the patient's chin, which closes the mouth and pulls the lower jaw anteriorly, relieving airway obstruction caused by the tongue. By positioning yourself at the patient's head during this maneuver, the palm of your hand is in close proximity to the nares; if there are spontaneous respirations, you can readily feel the patient's breath on your palm. These maneuvers also free the anesthesiologist's or surgeon's other hand to continue applying pressure to the now-anesthetized eye, if necessary.

Peribulbar Block

In this approach, the anesthetic is injected outside the muscle cone and allowed to diffuse inward. The advantage of the peribulbar injection is safety. Almost no risk of intrathecal anesthesia exists, and orbital hemorrhage and scleral perforation are much less likely than with a retrobulbar block; of particular concern when operating on eyes with long axial lengths. The chief disadvantages are a longer onset of action and a more frequent failure to achieve adequate anesthesia or akinesia. Adequate peribulbar blocks can require up to 8–10 ml of anesthetic, depending on orbital size, and can therefore cause significant proptosis and chemosis (White 1997).

In cases in which a peribulbar or retrobulbar block is used and orbicularis function is compromised, an occlusive eye patch is required to keep the eyelid closed. This prevents corneal trauma resulting from lagophthalmos secondary to orbicularis paresis. In addition, patch occlusion prevents binocular diplopia from extraocular muscle paresis.

Complications of Local Blocks

Chemosis

Isolated chemosis in the absence of a retrobulbar hemorrhage can occur if the anesthetic block is injected or diffuses into the subconjunctival space. Significant chemosis suggests that much of the anesthetic has not been injected into the muscle cone, which may result in suboptimal akinesia. A successful surgical outcome relies on the surgeon's ability to operate despite boggy conjunctival tissue, which can obscure the surgeon's view or impede surgical manipulations.

In the case of severe chemosis, a conjunctival incision to decompress the subconjunctival space may be of tremendous help.

Subconjunctival Hemorrhage

A subconjunctival hemorrhage not associated with a retrobulbar hemorrhage is of little consequence unless it is so severe that it results in marked elevation of the conjunctiva, which can obscure the surgeon's view or impede the manipulation of instruments.

Subconjunctival hemorrhages clear in 1–3 weeks as long as the patient avoids straining maneuvers, has normal blood pressure, and does not take aspirin or other anticoagulants.

Retrobulbar Hemorrhage

The key to managing a retrobulbar hemorrhage is early detection. The clinical signs include

1. Conjunctival chemosis with variable subconjunctival hemorrhage. Subconjunctival hemorrhage may be confined to one or two quadrants or may completely encircle the globe. As a general rule, the more severe the retrobulbar hemorrhage, the greater the amount of subconjunctival blood. Retrobulbar hemorrhage may be limited, however, especially if the diagnosis is suspected early and the measures described in the following section are taken.
2. Increased IOP, resulting in a very firm globe.
3. Increasing proptosis and resistance to retropulsion of the globe.
4. Variable ecchymosis near the injection site.

If there is limited retrobulbar hemorrhage with low or normal IOP, the operation can possibly proceed.

In the event of a severe retrobulbar hemorrhage with elevated IOP, consider the following:

1. Topical IOP-lowering medications.
2. Intermittent pressure with the palm of the hand: 45 seconds on, 15 seconds off.
3. Intravenous mannitol (0.5–1.0 g/kg). Observe the patient carefully for signs of congestive heart failure or hypotension.

Defer surgery if there is marked chemosis and subconjunctival hemorrhage or increased IOP. Continue observation and treatment until IOP is reduced to normal.

If IOP fails to decrease, perform a lateral canthotomy and if necessary, a cantholysis of the inferior portion of the lateral canthal tendon. Do not waste valuable time measuring IOP if the globe is clearly firm to palpation.

Globe Perforation

When inserting the needle for a retrobulbar or peribulbar block, it is important to gently oscillate the needle tip while watching the globe to ensure that the needle does not engage the sclera. In the event of intracameral injection after a single perforation, the globe may become either extremely firm or extremely soft.

If a globe perforation is discovered once the procedure is initiated, it may be prudent to complete the operation and then immediately obtain a retina consultation.

Intrathecal Injection

Injection of local anesthesia into the optic nerve sheath can have dire consequences. The signs and symptoms include

1. Dilation of the contralateral pupil
2. Uncontrollable shaking and tremors
3. Loss of consciousness
4. Unresponsiveness to verbal and painful stimuli
5. Loss of deep tendon reflexes
6. Initial hypertension followed by hypotension
7. Respiratory arrest

The presence of any of these signs, which typically occur 2–5 minutes after injection, strongly suggests an intrathecal injection of anesthetic. The patient should be observed, and respirations must be monitored and supported as necessary. Hypotension must be treated with intravenous vasoconstrictors. Surgery must be deferred until the patient becomes totally conscious and is breathing normally. Elevating the head, which allows gravity to redistribute the anesthetic in the subarachnoid space, promotes a faster recovery. Our experience reveals that in the majority of these patients, surgery can proceed as little as 20 minutes after the intrathecal injection.

Note that administration of regional (retrobulbar or peribulbar) anesthesia to a fully draped patient should be avoided, because draping may mask many of the signs and symptoms of an anesthetic complication. It is critically important to have unobstructed access to the patient's head, neck, and extremities during anesthetic administration.

Topical Anesthesia

Although local anesthetic blocks are quite safe and effective, topical anesthesia, in the hands of a skilled phacoemulsification surgeon, offers several distinct advantages:

1. Immediate visual rehabilitation
2. Virtually no systemic side effects
3. No risk of retrobulbar hemorrhage
4. No risk of globe perforation
5. No requirement for an eye patch
6. No requirement for traction suture (this decreases the risk of associated ptosis)
7. No anesthesia-induced diplopia or ptosis
8. No postoperative periorbital numbness or paresthesias

However, there are a number of disadvantages to topical anesthesia:

1. The surgery is more challenging, owing to saccadic eye movements during surgery.
2. Patients must be able to cooperate and follow directions regarding eye movement.
3. It may not be appropriate for extremely anxious patients, those with hearing disabilities, or those with language barriers.
4. The potential exists for more postoperative pain from prolonged procedures or from those involving iris manipulation.

Keep in mind that topically administered anesthetics drain into the nasal cavity via the nasolacrimal duct, and they may affect the pharynx, potentially resulting in airway compromise.

The key to maximizing success with topical anesthesia, especially initially, is proper patient selection. Topical anesthesia can be used with clear corneal or scleral incisions and is appropriate for phacoemulsification or extracapsular expression. Whether topical anesthesia provides the same level of patient comfort as infiltrative local blocks is controversial. Regarding topical anesthesia, some patients report that the bright light of the operating microscope causes significant discomfort, and others report that the sensitivity of their eyelids and periorbital skin contributes to discomfort and anxiety. Some patients experience discomfort from the use of wet-field cautery or movement of the lens or iris diaphragm. The eye movements that occur with topical anesthesia can be used to your advantage by asking the patient to gaze in the appropriate direction when making an incision, inserting the phacoemulsifier tip, or accessing the cortex, as this eliminates the need for a traction suture.

Topical Anesthesia Techniques

Sterile, preservative-free topical anesthetic agents, such as methylparaben-free 0.75% bupivacaine hydrochloride, should be used. Every attempt should be made to avoid applying the drop directly onto the cornea, as this can result in epithelial toxicity. Use a cellulose sponge to absorb any fluid in the conjunctival fornices before instilling the anesthetic drop; this prevents loss of effect from dilution. Application of the topical anesthetic in a circumlimbal pattern anesthetizes the long ciliary nerves while protecting the cornea. In some cases, intravenous sedation can be a useful adjunct to topical or intracameral anesthesia.

Intracameral Anesthesia

One percent methylparaben-free (unpreserved) lidocaine is an excellent adjunct to topical anesthesia (Koch 1997; Gills et al. 1997). A 0.25- to 0.50-ml bolus may be injected into the AC after creating the incision. Warn the patient in advance that a burning sensation may be felt as the anesthesia is injected. Intracameral anesthesia helps the patient tolerate the microscope light and reduces sensation in the ciliary body.

Regional Eyelid Blocks

O'Brien Block

The O'Brien block anesthetizes the superior branch of the seventh cranial nerve as it passes anterior to the tragus and deep to the maxillary condyle (O'Brien). This block is generally no longer recommended due to its potential to affect a wide spectrum of nontarget tissues (Schimek and Fahle 1995).

The disadvantages of the O'Brien block include

1. It requires considerable practice to learn.
2. There may be postoperative pain with jaw movement.
3. The risk of anesthetizing inferior branches of the facial nerve involving the lips and lower face.
4. The risk of injection into the temporomandibular joint.
5. The risk of injuring the facial nerve.
6. Potential injury to the parotid duct with resulting blood-tinged saliva.
7. The risk of injection into the external auditory canal (rare).

Van Lint Block

The anesthetic agent is infiltrated in the subcutaneous space in the vicinity of the temporal and buccinator branches of the seventh nerve (Van Lint 1914). This block is particularly useful when the patient is anxious and squeezes both eyes closed throughout the procedure.

The disadvantages of a Van Lint block include

1. Edema of the eyelids and ecchymosis
2. Pain with infiltration of soft tissues

Atkinson Block

In an Atkinson block, local anesthetic is infiltrated in the region of the lateral canthus. The Atkinson block is commonly used and is somewhat of a compromise between the Van Lint and O'Brien blocks (Atkinson 1953).

Nadbath (Retroauricular, Stylomastoid) Block

The Nadbath block (Figure 2-1) anesthetizes the main trunk of the facial nerve. The injection is placed at the anteroinferior margin of the concavity in the skin inferior to the external auditory meatus. The needle is directed perpendicular to the skin (Nadbath and Rehman 1963). We recommend using

Figure 2-1. Retroauricular block.

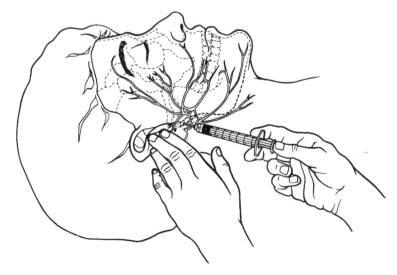

2 ml of anesthetic with epinephrine. Do not use hyaluronidase for this block.

The disadvantages of a Nadbath block include

1. The risk of intravascular injection.
2. The risk of involvement of the muscles of mastication and depression of the swallowing reflex due to spread of the block, which can lead to choking on endogenous secretions.
3. The risk of lip droop.
4. It must be avoided in stroke patients with contralateral facial weakness, because of the potential involvement of the muscles of swallowing.

Severe asthma, chronic obstructive pulmonary disease (COPD) with thick pharyngeal secretions, and the patient's use of the accessory muscles of respiration are all contraindications of a Nadbath block.

Retroauricular blocks are generally not recommended, because they block a wide range of non-target tissues.

General Anesthesia Techniques

With the advent of less intrusive surgical techniques (small incision surgery), and the variety of regional and topical anesthetic options, general anesthesia is rarely used in cataract surgery and should be reserved for special circumstances in which patient cooperation is impossible (e.g., pediatric cases, adults with significant tremors). The clear advantages of general anesthesia include absolute immobilization of the head and globe and complete absence of sensation and recall. The concomitant administration of retrobulbar or peribulbar regional blocks may reduce general anesthesia dosing requirements and promote postoperative comfort. Disadvantages of general anesthesia include serious systemic risks, prolonged postoperative recovery, gastrointestinal side effects, and considerable cost.

It is not our intent here to discuss the complex art of administering general anesthesia. The intubation techniques and the agents used are determined by the anesthesiologist. Nevertheless, it is the surgeon's responsibility to express preferences and goals to the anesthesiologist and provide an estimate of the procedure's duration.

Some practical aspects of general anesthesia are of considerable importance to the surgeon. Placement of the endotracheal tube should not interfere with proper ophthalmic draping or subsequent surgical maneuvers. The endotracheal tube should be of low profile and positioned on the side of the mouth contralateral to the surgical eye to minimize the risk of jostling and disconnection from the anesthesia circuit. Using a narrow endotracheal extension tube with a connector creates a relatively unobstructed surgical field. An oral RAE endotracheal tube, which has a preformed, low-profile curve, is an excellent choice for general anesthesia.

Chapter 3
Instrumentation and Equipment

Required Instruments and Supplies

The operating room should be furnished with the following elements (or their equivalents):

1. Full-body or partial drape
2. Plastic eye drape without aperture
3. Steri-Strips
4. Wire-lid speculum
5. Self-retaining speculum
6. Fenestrated aspirating speculum
7. Fine-Thornton fixating ring
8. Toothed forceps (0.12)
9. Diamond or stainless-steel keratome
10. Diamond or stainless-steel crescent blade
11. No. 6400 or No. 6900 Beaver blade
12. 15-Degree disposable blade
13. Capsulorhexis forceps
14. Cystotome
15. Bent 25-gauge needle
16. Westcott scissors
17. Vannas scissors
18. Sinskey hook
19. Kuglen hook
20. Lester hook
21. Nucleus chopper
22. Nucleus cracker
23. Cyclodialysis spatula
24. Topical proparacaine (0.5%)
25. Preservative-free lidocaine 1%
26. Balanced salt solution (BSS)
27. Epinephrine (1:2,000)
28. Vancomycin (1 mg/ml)
29. Nylon sutures (9-0 and 10-0)
30. Needle holder
31. Tying forceps
32. Kratz capsule scraper
33. Terry Squeegee (Alcon Surgical Inc., Fort Worth, TX)
34. Muscle hook
35. Lens loop
36. Endocapsular ring
37. Lens loop amputator
38. Hand-held cylindrical keratoscope
39. Banked scleral tissue

Operating Table

The ideal operating table includes a headrest that can be adjusted in all directions and firmly fixed once properly positioned. An adjustable headrest allows greater flexibility in head and neck positioning, permitting the surgeon to precisely position the operative eye. The table should tilt, allowing the patient to be placed in the Fowler or Trendelenburg positions, and lateral tilting should be possible as well. The table should consist of sections that permit flexion at the hips and knees to maximize the patient's comfort.

In surgery centers catering primarily to ambulatory patients, an electric reclining chair similar to a dentist's chair helps maximize the patient's comfort and decreases turnaround time, as the patient can simply walk to and from the chair with ease.

Surgical Microscope

A wide variety of quality surgical microscopes is available. The microscope should include the following features:

1. Strong, uniform, coaxial lighting that allows a clear red reflex
2. X-Y axis foot pedal control
3. A range of zoom magnification levels
4. An observer microscope with binocular, and preferably coaxial, view
5. Option for a video camera and simultaneous observer microscope

Many surgical microscopes incorporate assistant microscopes that have only a noncoaxial monocular view. This puts the assistant or observer at a disadvantage, because the anterior and posterior capsules may be indiscernible with such limited optical devices.

When using a video camera, a one-chip model is adequate for clear images. A three-chip model is much more expensive but allows higher resolution.

It is convenient to have an eclipse feature or a differential central-lighting system whereby portions of the operative field can be only dimly lit to help prevent macular phototoxicity during some steps of the surgery, such as wound suturing.

When positioning the microscope, start high above the patient's head, center the microscope over the operative eye, and move the microscope downward toward the globe until the corneal apex begins to appear in clear focus. Using the fine adjustment to focus from the corneal apex to the iris prevents accommodation.

If you are using a video camera, focus the image on the video monitor first, then independently adjust the focus on the microscope oculars to create a sharp view.

Magnification

Use of very high magnification can stimulate accommodation, making it difficult to keep the surgical area within the microscopic field. The higher the magnification, the more difficult the centering and focusing of the image. Inadequately low magnification may prevent the visualization of subtle capsular contours or opacities adhering to the posterior capsule.

Lighting

Once the microscope is illuminating the field and an adequate red reflex is obtained, the overhead and ceiling lights of the operating room should be turned off. The reduction of ambient light enhances the contrast in the operating field, making it easier to visualize the lens capsule, nucleus, and cortex. The scrub nurse should have access to a focal spotlight for illumination of the Mayo instrument stand.

Keratometers

Cataract surgeons vary with respect to their use of intraoperative keratometry. Its low accuracy and reliability may limit its clinical benefit. Although intraoperative corneal topography is of some interest, the results that become apparent in the weeks and months after surgery are more clinically significant. The effects of wound healing vary widely among patients and can be large; a spheric intraoperative corneal surface does not guarantee a spheric surface several weeks later.

Phacoemulsifier

The development of phacoemulsification by Charles Kelman (Kelman 1967) revolutionized cataract surgery and instrumentation. Several different phacoemulsification systems are available, and many others are sure to be introduced. The basic principles of irrigation, phacoemulsifier power, and aspiration are similar across all systems, but significant differences in fluidics do exist.

Venturi pump systems work on the principle of vacuum created by rapid flow streams, whereas peristaltic systems depend on a revolving roller that squeezes the tubing to create fluid flow. Relatively sophisticated systems exist that can change aspiration flow rate and vacuum parameters at the instant total lumen occlusion occurs, reducing the risk of posterior capsular rupture during a postocclusion surge.

If possible, confine your surgical cases to one surgical center or at least to one phacoemulsification system. If you must use different phacoemulsification systems, learn the nuances and idiosyncrasies of each system before attempting your first case.

Many phacoemulsification units allow multiple surgeons to each store their preferred power, vacuum, and aspiration settings. Make the effort to determine and store the parameters that work best for you.

Infusion Bottle

A sterile BSS (Sterile Irrigating Solution, Alcon Laboratories Inc., Fort Worth, TX) should be used for infusion during surgery. A combination of antibiotics, such as vancomycin and gentamicin, may be added to provide gram-positive and gram-negative coverage. Keep in mind that intraocular gentamicin carries a risk of irreversible macular toxicity, and that the benefits of adding antibiotics to the irrigation fluid are controversial. The use of mydriatic agents, however, such as 0.5 ml of 1:1,000 epinephrine added to the 500-ml BSS bottle, is quite effective in maintaining a dilated pupil (Corbett and Richards 1994) and is well tolerated systemically (Fiore and Cinotti 1988).

Viscoelastics

Numerous viscoelastic agents, each with their own purported benefits, are available. Most viscoelastic agents consist of 1% sodium hyaluronate (10 mg/ml). Viscoelastics fall into one of two general categories: cohesive and adhesive (or dispersive).

Cohesive viscoelastics, as the name implies, tend to be self-adherent. Consequently, they can be easily removed from the AC. They are easily removed at the end of surgery and therefore less likely to result in a postoperative IOP spike, but offer little protection to the corneal endothelium because they are easily removed by aspiration at the phacoemulsifier tip.

Adhesive viscoelastics, on the other hand, tend to adhere to ocular structures. Consequently, they tend to coat the endothelium and offer a protective effect during surgery. However, they are difficult to remove at the end of surgery. Considerable irrigation-aspiration flow and time are required to remove these viscoelastics from the AC.

Neodymium:yttrium-aluminum Garnet Laser

Having a neodymium:yttrium-aluminum garnet (Nd:YAG) laser near the operating suite can be very useful in certain cases. As explained in Chapters 12 and 14, the preoperative creation of an anterior capsular opening with a laser can greatly increase the likelihood of a favorable outcome.

Chapter 4
Preoperative Preparations

Although meticulous surgical technique is essential for achieving a successful result, attention to a variety of factors before surgery can greatly enhance the final outcome.

Pupillary Dilatation

Wide dilatation of the pupil before surgery is essential. The surgeon should start by producing the maximum pharmacologic dilatation possible. This is best accomplished using a combination of a sympathetic agonist and a parasympathetic antagonist. For most cases, 2.5% topical phenylephrine combined with 0.5% tropicamide is quite effective for maintaining a widely dilated pupil. In patients with pseudoexfoliation or a history of chronic miotic-agent use, 10% phenylephrine may be helpful. Ideally, these eyedrops should be placed in the operative eye at least an hour before surgery. It may be helpful to have the patient use these eye drops at home, before coming to the operating room. Repeating the dosage two or three times at 10- to 15-minute intervals may enhance the dilation. Remember that topical sympathomimetic agents drain via the nasolacrimal duct, allowing systemic absorption across the nasal mucosa and potentially resulting in a hypertensive crisis. The preoperative use of NSAIDs may also prevent miosis during cataract surgery, especially if the procedure is prolonged or involves iris manipulation or trauma (Cillino et al. 1993). As your level of skill increases, the routine use of NSAIDs becomes largely unnecessary.

Nonpreserved epinephrine, 0.5 ml (1:1,000), can be added to the 500-ml infusion bottle of BSS to maintain a dilated pupil throughout the case (Corbett and Richards 1994), as discussed in Chapter 3. During surgery, 0.25 ml of intraocular epinephrine (1:2,000) may be injected into the AC to facilitate pharmacologic dilation of the pupil. Unlike topical phenylephrine, intraocular epinephrine is not absorbed systemically, so there is no effect on systemic blood pressure. Additionally, if methylparaben-free 1% intracameral lidocaine is used, this also has an intrinsic pupil-dilating effect (Hsu et al. 1999).

Surgical methods of dilating the pupil are discussed in Chapter 12.

Preoperative Intraocular Pressure

If extracapsular nuclear expression is planned, a soft eye at the outset of surgery reduces the likelihood of an expulsive choroidal hemorrhage. Such hemorrhages are quite rare in small-incision phacoemulsification surgery owing to the closed system maintained for most of the surgery. The importance of a soft eye before cataract surgery is often overstated. Nonetheless, a low IOP at the start of surgery decreases the chances of expulsive suprachoroidal hemorrhage, iris prolapse, and vitreous prolapse, and helps maintain a deep AC throughout the operation.

Situations in which lowering IOP should be considered include

- Patients younger than 50 years (who have formed vitreous humor)
- Patients with a history of positive vitreous pressure during cataract surgery on the fellow eye
- Elderly hypertensive patients who are at risk for an expulsive choroidal hemorrhage
- A significantly elevated IOP at the start of surgery

Methods of Lowering Preoperative Intraocular Pressure

Intermittent Digital Pressure

When intermittent digital pressure is used to lower IOP, the fingertips are used to push on the globe episodically. Pressure is applied to a gauze pad placed over the closed upper eyelid for approximately 20 seconds, then is withdrawn for 10 seconds. This is repeated for several minutes as necessary until the globe is soft. Ballottement may be used to assess IOP. The use of a tonometer to assess IOP during surgery is generally unnecessary and adds the risk of corneal abrasion.

Mercury Bags and Honan Balloons

Practically no need exists for mercury bags or Honan balloons in small-incision surgery. In rare cases in which the risk of expulsive choroidal hemorrhage is high (e.g., when there is a history of expulsive choroidal hemorrhage in the fellow eye), these devices may be helpful.

A mercury bag allows the application of constant pressure through the placement of a known weight on the closed eyelid. A Honan balloon is a pneumatic pressure device that can be applied to the eye using a rubber strap encircling the head. Gauze padding of sufficient thickness should be placed between the closed eyelid and the Honan balloon to evenly distribute the balloon's pressure. Care should be taken to ensure that the balloon pressure does not exceed 30 mm Hg, as measured by an attached pressure gauge. Although Honan balloons can be helpful in certain settings, they are difficult to apply and must be monitored quite carefully because they

can slide into an improper position with even the slightest movement by the patient.

Any IOP-lowering method involving mechanical pressure on the globe carries the potential risk of ischemic optic neuropathy. Elevated IOP can decrease the blood flow to the choroidal and retinal circulations as well as anterior segment, potentially resulting in ischemic damage to ocular structures, especially the optic nerve, which may be irreversibly damaged. Intermittently elevated IOP of short duration is unlikely to cause as much damage as prolonged exposure to high pressure; however, the potential risk of ischemic damage from any of these methods should be kept in mind. Ischemic damage sustained by an already compromised nerve may be catastrophic.

Acetazolamide

Acetazolamide is a carbonic anhydrase inhibitor that reduces aqueous production. It is contraindicated in renal failure, sulfa allergies, and electrolyte imbalances. There have been reports of aplastic anemia and Stevens-Johnson syndrome from acetazolamide. Although it does not reduce vitreous volume, acetazolamide may be useful to prevent postoperative IOP spikes.

Mannitol

Mannitol is extremely effective for relatively rapid dehydration of the vitreous. Patients with COPD, for example, often have venous congestion, resulting in elevations of IOP.

Mannitol may also be useful in cases of expulsive or threatened choroidal hemorrhage. As this condition may result in acute hypertension, blood pressure should be carefully monitored during mannitol administration. Care should be taken when using mannitol because of its significant systemic effects, however, especially in patients with congestive heart failure. Mannitol can cause hypertension, diuresis, and rebound hypotension.

Mannitol may be contraindicated in congestive heart failure, renal failure, severe prostatic disease (owing to obstructive urinary retention) and in pediatric patients. Careful monitoring of vital signs during dosing is essential. If mannitol administration is planned, ask the patient to void just before arriving in the operating room. In rare prolonged cases using general anesthesia, mannitol's diuretic effect may require urinary catheterization of the patient during surgery. A dose of 0.5–1.0 g/kg, rather than the 2 g/kg often recommended, is generally adequate. The infusion should be started once the patient arrives in the preoperative holding area to allow sufficient time before the start of surgery.

Oral Osmotic Diuretics

Oral osmotic diuretics, such as isosorbide, although quite effective in lowering IOP, are generally contraindicated preoperatively because of a high incidence of nausea and especially vomiting, which can lead to aspiration.

Positioning the Patient

Many surgeons overlook the importance of proper patient positioning before the start of surgery. Although it may seem simple, the proper positioning of the patient during surgery is critical to surgical success. It is important for both patient and surgeon to be as comfortable as possible throughout the procedure. As most cataract patients are elderly, they often have musculoskeletal abnormalities, such as kyphosis, scoliosis, and arthritis, that require careful positioning of the back and extremities. Improvisation is critical to ensure the comfort of the patient.

For example, simply propping a pillow under the patient's knees allows more relaxing flexion of these joints. Similarly, a rolled towel or bed sheet under the lower back can supply lumbar support if necessary.

The torso's position can be as important as the head's. The body should be inclined in the Fowler's (reversed Trendelenburg) position, as this enhances venous drainage away from the head and neck, lowering IOP. This posture also alleviates pressure of the abdominal contents on the diaphragm, making breathing more comfortable.

The headrest should be carefully adjusted so the plane of the iris is parallel to the floor. It may be useful to use the chin and forehead as landmarks to maintain a horizontal plane (Figure 4-1A). The microscope light should be perpendicular to this plane and a good red reflex should be obtained through the pupil. Any deviation from this can compromise the red reflex and place the surgeon's hands in an awkward position during manipulation of the lenticular nucleus (Figures 4-1B and 4-1C). When operating superiorly, it may actually be necessary to raise the patient's chin slightly higher than the forehead, depending on the prominence of the patient's brow.

Surgeon's Position

Although the patient's comfort is critical during surgery, the surgeon's positioning is equally impor-

Figure 4-1. A. Proper head tilt. **B.** Head tilt with chin too high; the patient's neck is uncomfortably hyperextended and the angle for the surgeon is awkward. Note that raising the chin *slightly* may be necessary for the superior approach in a patient with a prominent brow. **C.** Head tilt with chin too low. The red reflex is compromised, and the brow becomes an obstacle if the incision is placed superiorly.

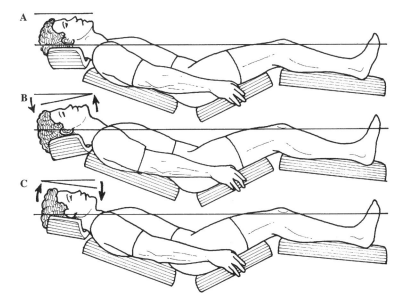

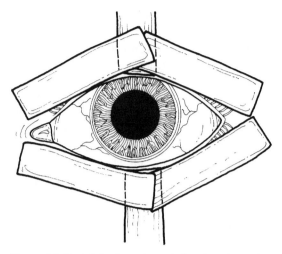

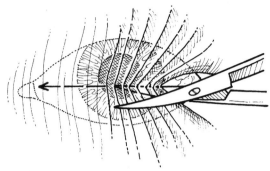

Figure 4-3. Creating a linear aperture in a clear drape.

Figure 4-2. Steri-Strips keep the eyelashes draped out of the operative field.

tant. Avoid a hunched-over posture, which stresses the lower back and neck. Your head should be evenly balanced on your neck, and your spine should be maintained in an erect, comfortable alignment. The foot pedals should be comfortably placed and your knees bent at right angles.

Sterile Skin Preparation

Meticulous care during sterile preparation is essential for preventing postoperative endophthalmitis. The vast majority of pathogens causing postoperative endophthalmitis arise from the endogenous flora of the eyelids and lashes. A carefully applied coat of povidone-iodine should be applied to the eyelids, lashes and surrounding facial skin. The povidone-iodine should first be applied to the lashes using a scrubbing motion, and then the povidone-iodine swab or gauze should be applied in concentric circles of increasing radius. The skin around the lids should be cleaned in an ever-expanding spiral, so that the eyebrows and nose are scrubbed last. The same pattern should be repeated two or three times using new povidone-iodine-soaked swaps. The povidone-iodine should remain on the skin for at least 2–3 minutes for maximal bactericidal effect. Excess povidone-iodine may then be carefully wiped away to promote adhesion of self-adhesive drapes. An alcohol swab may be applied in the same pattern to remove povidone-iodine stains.

Sterile gauze should be used to wipe any alcohol from the skin, so the adhesive drapes can adhere more firmly.

Perhaps the most useful adjunct in the prevention of postoperative infection is a topical 5% povidone-iodine solution containing 0.5% available iodine (Speaker and Menicoff 1991). After the instillation of topical anesthetic into the conjunctiva (with care taken to avoid the central cornea), one to two drops of topical povidone-iodine should be instilled onto the cornea and allowed to spread across the bulbar conjunctiva and conjunctival cul-de-sacs. The topical povidone-iodine should be irrigated with sterile BSS solution 1–2 minutes later.

Draping

A forehead drape is used in combination with a body drape to cover uninvolved areas of the operative field. Adhesive tape, such as Steri-Strips (3M Health Care, Borken, Germany), should be used to retract the lids. The tape should be placed near the base of the eyelashes to ensure that all lashes are draped out of the surgical field (Figure 4-2). A clear plastic drape may then be placed over the globe and lids. The advantage of using a drape without a pre-existing aperture is that the lashes and lid margins can be completely covered without tedious placement of the adhesive drape. In some cases, this technique of draping can eliminate the need for a lid speculum. Be sure that the drapes lift the eyelids away from the globe rather than exert pressure on the eye. Carefully incise a linear opening in the clear plastic drape while pulling it anteriorly, away from the cornea (Figure 4-3).

Lid Speculum

The lid speculum should retract the eyelids for optimal globe exposure while remaining unobtrusive. Speculums with a cross bar, although quite sturdy, should be avoided because this bar severely restricts the movement of the phacoemulsifier tip when the surgeon operates superiorly. A wire, Kratz-style speculum retracts the lids very well while still allowing free movement of the phacoemulsifier handpiece.

In some cases, the patient's lid anatomy and head tilt allow pooling of topically instilled BSS in the medial canthus and submerges the cornea in fluid, obscuring the surgeon's view. Recognizing this fluid collection early in surgery and taking appropriate measures prevents unnecessary complications. If fluid pooling occurs, the simplest solution is to tilt the patient's head laterally toward the operative eye. If this results in poor positioning for the surgeon, a collagen wick can be placed at least 5 mm into the lateral canthus to absorb the fluid pool. Alternatively, a fenestrated speculum can be attached to gentle wall suction or a 60-ml syringe to aspirate fluid that pools on the ocular surface.

Superior Rectus Traction Suture

Clear corneal phacoemulsification with topical anesthesia makes a traction suture unnecessary. For a scleral tunnel procedure using a local block, a superior rectus traction suture is optional to tort the globe inferiorly for a 12:00 approach. This has the advantage of exposing the superior limbus and allowing comfortable positioning to create any type of incision.

Placement of the Superior Rectus Traction Suture

The following steps describe the technique used in the placement of a superior rectus traction suture.

1. Using two sets of closed forceps, tort the globe into infraduction using a hand-over-hand technique. Grasping the conjunctiva with the jaws of the forceps results in better control, but may cause subconjunctival hemorrhage and trauma to the conjunctiva.

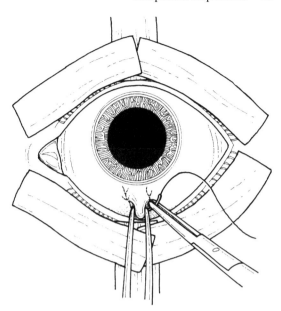

Figure 4-4. Placing a superior rectus traction suture.

2. Identify the insertion of the superior rectus tendon through the conjunctiva and Tenon's fascia.
3. Use a toothed forceps to grasp the conjunctiva, Tenon's fascia, and superior rectus tendon, just superior to the latter's insertion into the globe.
4. Pass a tapered or cardiovascular needle through the tendon just posterior to the tips of the grasping forceps, being careful not to penetrate the globe (Figure 4-4). A bite that is too superficial results in inadequate traction on the globe, whereas one that is too deep results in scleral penetration or perforation.

Superior Rectus Traction Suture Risks

1. Ptosis, secondary to trauma to the levator palpebrae superioris or its innervation.
2. Diplopia, secondary to trauma to the superior rectus.
3. Subconjunctival hemorrhage or superior rectus muscle hematoma.
4. Globe perforation, because the suture is passed without direct visualization.

Chapter 5
Incisions

The incision is one of the most critical components of surgery. The quality of the incision affects the ease of nuclear removal, the implantation of the IOL, the postoperative visual outcome, and the risk of infection.

Scleral Tunnel Incision

A self-sealing scleral tunnel incision creates a very stable wound that can be constructed to induce varying amounts of corneal steepening or flattening in the incision meridian. A wide variety of incision lengths are possible; these range from 2 mm to 6 clock-hours. The key to successful scleral wound construction is creating sharp, smooth edges to avoid a ragged incision margin.

Conjunctival Flap

A conjunctival flap is necessary for the construction of a scleral incision. The technique for creating a fornix-based conjunctival flap is as follows:

1. Grasp the bulbar conjunctiva just posterior to the limbus using a smooth forceps and tent anteriorly into a fold perpendicular to the limbus.
2. Using sharp Westcott scissors, make a small snip at the fold creating a small incision parallel to the limbus.
3. Insert the closed Westcott scissors subconjunctivally, parallel to the limbus and along the path of the planned incision.
4. Open the blades of the scissors, bluntly separating the potential subconjunctival plane (Figure 5-1).
5. Incise the conjunctiva at its insertion along the length of the incision, pulling the scissor blades anteriorly to cut along the limbus (Figure 5-2). The conjunctival incision should be slightly longer than the planned scleral incision.
6. Repeat this undermining and cutting until the appropriate incision length is reached. For extracapsular cataract expression, expose slightly less than one-half of the superior limbus; for phacoemulsification, expose 4–7 mm of limbal area, depending on the IOL to be used. When making the conjunctival incision, avoid jagged edges and residual ruffles on the conjunctiva at the limbus. If a nubbin of conjunctival tissue remains at the limbus, either remove it by scraping with a Beaver (Visitec, Sarasota, FL; Becton Dickinson, Franklin Lakes, NJ) No. 6900 blade or excise it using Westcott or Vannas scissors.
7. Repeat these steps to incise Tenon's fascia at its insertion.
8. Cauterize episcleral vessels lightly with wet-field cautery using a coaxial bipolar tip or McPherson forceps adapted for this purpose. Avoid excessive cautery to prevent charring and contraction

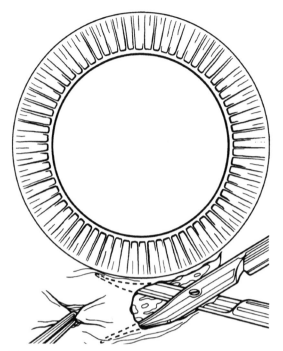

Figure 5-1. Spreading open scissor blades for a blunt dissection.

of scleral fibers, which can induce corneal steepening. Start with the lowest cautery setting and gradually increase until the desired effect is achieved.

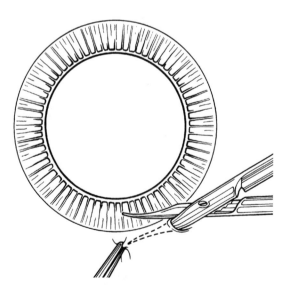

Figure 5-2. Pull the scissor blades anteriorly to incise at the conjunctival insertion.

Comments

A fornix-based conjunctival flap can be used for extracapsular cataract extraction, phacoemulsification, or combined cataract extraction and trabeculectomy. A conjunctival incision should not be used if a filtering bleb is present or if there is excessive scarring, such as from the peritomy for a scleral-buckling procedure.

In elderly patients with thin Tenon's fascia, the conjunctiva and Tenon's fascia may be undermined and incised together in one flap. In younger patients, it may be useful to perform the dissections separately to create smoother incision edges and for anatomic closure in layers at the end of surgery. Fibrotic ridges can occur from a poorly constructed incision as the conjunctival flap scars postoperatively, and these disruptions in the normally smooth ocular surface can cause irritation and discontinuities in the tear film.

Constructing the Scleral Tunnel

Once the appropriate conjunctival incision is made, proceed with the scleral incision:

1. Fix the globe using toothed forceps or a fixation ring.
2. Incise a partial-thickness scleral groove 1–2 mm posterior to the limbal arcades, parallel to the limbus, with a Beaver No. 6900 or No. 6400 blade (Figure 5-3). The depth of this groove should be one-half to two-thirds of scleral thickness.
3. Dissect a lamellar scleral tunnel using an angled crescent blade, staying parallel to the scleral plane.
4. Extend the dissection laterally to the ends of the initial groove and anteriorly to incorporate 1 mm of clear cornea.
5. As you advance centrally, you must tilt the leading edge of the blade anteriorly to follow the convex curvature of the peripheral cornea (Figure 5-4) to prevent premature entry into the AC.
6. Gently slide a keratome of appropriate width into the scleral tunnel at the midpoint of your incision. Use a light side-to-side motion to help guide the keratome into the proper plane. Advance the keratome, without cutting, until resistance is met at the central extent of your dissection (Figure 5-5).

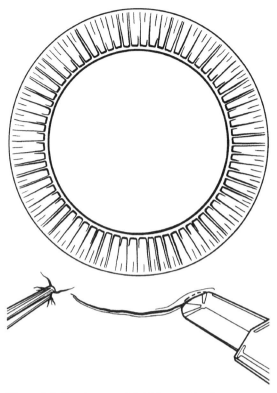

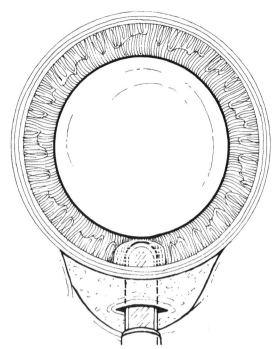

Figure 5-4. Tunnel into the clear cornea, being careful to angle the tip of the blade anteriorly as the corneal convexity is approached.

Figure 5-3. Creating a partial-thickness scleral groove.

7. Angle the tip of the keratome posteriorly and enter the AC with a smooth incising motion, creating a beveled entry and preventing the stripping of Descemet's membrane. A Descemet's detachment is more likely to occur if the keratome is advanced nearly parallel to the plane of the endothelium.

Comments

It is helpful to limit the width of the scleral tunnel dissection to that required for the phacoemulsifier tip rather than that needed for the IOL. The intact sclera adjacent to the incision affords strength, preventing the tearing of Descemet's membrane during phacoemulsification and cortical removal.

Creating a 6-mm scleral tunnel before phacoemulsification may result in dehiscence of the smaller internal wound, resulting in excessive outflow of irrigation fluid, collapse of the AC, or iris prolapse.

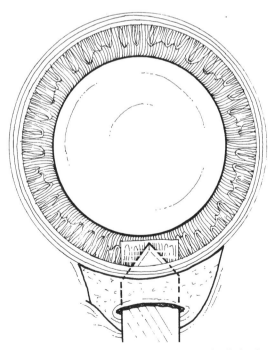

Figure 5-5. Advance the keratome to the anterior limit of the sclerocorneal tunnel before cutting any tissue to maintain a smooth dissection plane.

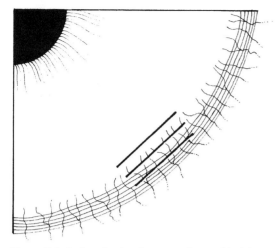

Figure 5-6. Options for the placement of corneal incisions.

Pros and Cons

The advantages of the scleral tunnel incision include (1) minimal corneal edema from the incision itself, (2) the reduction of postoperative astigmatism, and (3) minimized postoperative irritation owing to the conjunctiva's covering of the incision and any sutures. The potential disadvantages include (1) conjunctival scarring, (2) ballooning of the conjunctiva by irrigation fluid, (3) intraoperative bleeding from scleral vessels, and (4) postoperative hyphemas.

Corneal Incisions

Corneal incisions differ from scleral incisions in a number of ways:

1. They are easier to construct.
2. They are essentially avascular, especially advantageous in patients with bleeding diatheses.
3. The potential for greater astigmatic effects exists.
4. More resistant to stretching.
5. No conjunctival scarring occurs, therefore preserving the conjunctiva for future glaucoma surgery.
6. Manipulation of pre-existing filtering blebs or glaucoma drainage devices is avoided (Park).

Corneal incisions are excellent for phacoemulsification using foldable IOLs and topical anesthesia.

The incisions are usually placed in clear cornea just anterior to the limbal arcades.

Uniplanar Clear Corneal Incision

Corneal incisions can be created quickly, do not require conjunctival manipulation, and seal more rapidly than their scleral counterparts. If a uniplanar corneal incision is made carefully and smooth edges are created, a watertight seal results from the "internal valve" effect of the cornea. Clear corneal incisions may be created anterior to, at, or posterior to the limbal arcades (Figure 5-6). For relatively inexperienced surgeons, it may be helpful to construct the incision anteriorly to reduce iris prolapse. A relatively anterior inner-incision lip is also useful in eyes with shallow ACs and narrow angles.

An incision created anterior to the limbal arcades (within the clear cornea) has the advantage of a truly avascular location and eliminates all bleeding complications from the incision site. The disadvantage of this approach is that it is most likely to result in induced astigmatic effects. If you are operating on the steep corneal meridian, the flattening produced by this incision may be advantageous; recognizing, however, that the effects may not be entirely predictable.

An incision made at the limbal arcades results in the greatest potential for incisional bleeding, but results in fewer astigmatic effects than a more anterior incision because of its more peripheral approach.

An incision made posterior to the limbal arcades has the least potential for incision-induced astigmatic effects. Because of its proximity to the conjunctival insertion, however, it may result in subconjunctival hemorrhage or ballooning of the conjunctiva secondary to irrigation fluid.

The procedure for the creation of a uniplanar clear corneal incision is as follows:

1. Use a 0.12 Bonn forceps or a fixation ring to maintain sufficient counterpressure for a controlled incision.
2. A stainless steel or diamond keratome may be used.
3. Introduce the point of the keratome at the desired location to create the posterior lip of the incision.
4. Slowly introduce the blade into the AC, angling it toward the corneal apex.

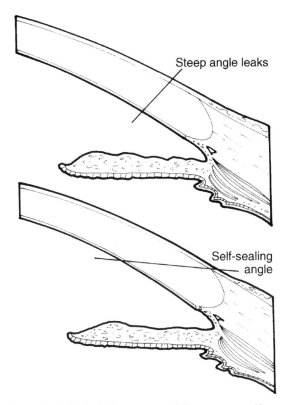

Figure 5-7. Angle the keratome carefully to create a self-sealing incision.

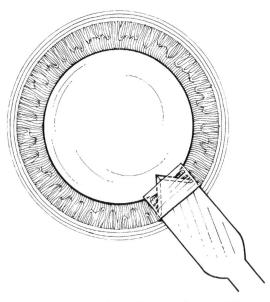

Figure 5-8. Withdrawal of the keratome from a uniplanar clear corneal incision.

The angle of the blade is extremely important in determining the manner in which tissues are apposed in wound closure. If the blade is held perpendicular to the surface of the cornea, the wound does not seal spontaneously because no valve is created (Figure 5-7). If the blade is placed tangential to the corneal curve, it does not enter the AC. Descemet's membrane may be stripped if the tip of the keratome is too anterior. For optimal incision construction, angle the tip of the keratome toward the corneal apex rather than parallel to the iris plane. Remember that because of the length of the handle, a large movement by your hand results in only a small change in the angle of the keratome blade. Withdraw the keratome in exactly the same plane used for entry (Figure 5-8).

Triplanar Clear Corneal Incision

A more stable corneal incision can be constructed by creating what is essentially a clear corneal tunnel (Figure 5-9). Creating a triplanar corneal wound allows you to make a large (7-mm) self-sealing incision that may not require sutures. Sutureless wounds of this length are not possible with a uniplanar corneal incision.

The procedure for creating a triplanar corneal incision is as follows:

1. Use a guarded diamond blade to create a partial-thickness corneal groove along the limbus at one-third to one-half of corneal depth.
2. Create a 1–2 mm corneal tunnel with an angled crescent blade.
3. Slide a keratome into this tunnel until resistance is met.

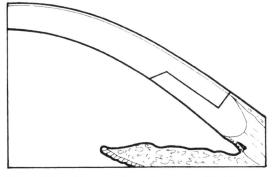

Figure 5-9. Architecture of a triplanar corneal incision.

4. Dimple posteriorly, angling the keratome and enter the AC.

Keratomes

Diamond versus Stainless Steel

Using a high-quality diamond blade results in very smooth incision edges, which promote a watertight seal. Diamond keratomes are, however, fragile and expensive, requiring meticulous care and trained personnel to preserve the blades in optimum condition. The blade should be advanced beyond its protective sheath only when making an incision. Because the exquisitely sharp edge of a diamond blade cuts tissue with minimal pressure, great care should be taken to prevent damage to tissues through the use of excessive force when creating or enlarging incisions.

Stainless-steel keratomes have the clear advantage of being more durable and affordable than diamond blades. A discernible difference in incision quality exists, however, especially if the stainless-steel blade is used more than once. Furthermore, blade edges vary from one to the next, although many modern steel keratomes are quite well designed and capable of creating excellent self-sealing incisions.

Acute versus Obtuse Blade Angles

The smaller the angle at the keratome tip, the sharper the blade. However, a blade with a very narrow-angled tip requires greater advancement into the AC to achieve the same incision width as a keratome with a wide-angled tip. The further the keratome is pushed into the AC, the greater the risk of damage to the anterior capsule or central corneal endothelium from the advancing tip.

Incision Location

Regardless of the type of incision—corneal or scleral—selected, the surgeon must decide on the location of the wound. Incision location can affect patient comfort and the amount of postoperative astigmatism. As a general rule, superior incisions remain covered by the upper eyelid and may be more comfortable than those made within the palpebral fissures. Realize, however, that a poorly constructed incision resulting in an uneven surface and irregular tear film may be uncomfortable in any location, whereas a properly constructed wound of any size or location may be quite comfortable.

Depending on the construction and closure of the incision, a cataract wound may induce either steepening or flattening along the incision meridian. Astigmatism resulting from cataract surgery can be attributed to (1) preoperative corneal astigmatism; (2) wound-induced changes in corneal curvature; and (3) IOL tilt, though this is a rare cause.

If a patient's preoperative corneal astigmatism is less than 0.50 diopters, an astigmatically neutral wound should be constructed, preferably temporally or posterior to the limbus to minimize its effect on central corneal curvature.

Corneal steepening along the wound meridian may be induced by using compression sutures. Flattening may be induced by constructing a long, sutureless, scleral tunnel wound.

Incision Size

Because incision size is influenced by surgical technique and the design of the proposed IOL implant, these factors should be considered when planning the surgery. For phacoemulsification cases, the initial incision (before it is enlarged for the IOL) should be long enough to accommodate the phacoemulsification needle but short enough to prevent excessive leakage of fluid and AC collapse. A true watertight seal around the phacoemulsifier's silicone sleeve makes it difficult to maneuver the phacoemulsifier tip and may result in a corneal burn unless a MacKool tip is used.

Side-Port Incisions

For two-handed phacoemulsification or irrigation-aspiration techniques, a clear corneal side port is necessary. However, many surgeons construct this incision less carefully than the main incision. The side-port incision should be as small as possible while still accommodating the intended instrument. Because these incisions are generally 1 mm or less, a uniplanar incision is sufficient for a watertight seal, provided the incision is angled slightly toward the corneal apex (Figure 5-10). Making a side-port incision parallel to the iris plane or angled toward the posterior pole often results in leakage during surgery and a poor seal afterwards. Owing to their small size, side-port incisions, once created, may be difficult to identify. It may be advantageous to place the incision within the limbal arcades, so that blood from the cut limbal capillaries can serve as a marker for the side-port site.

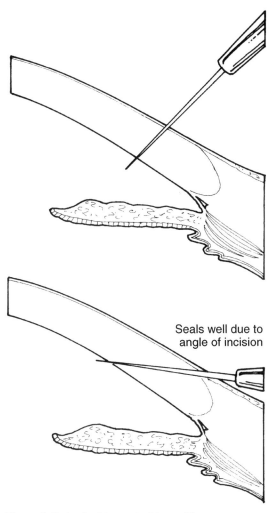

Figure 5-10. Angle side-port incisions with care to promote self-sealing.

Chapter 6
Anterior Capsular Opening, Hydrodissection, and Hydrodelineation

Before creating disruptions in the anterior lens capsule, the AC should be stabilized using a viscoelastic in a closed system. If no viscoelastic is available, an AC maintainer attached to gravity-driven irrigation may be used. The surgeon should concentrate on maintaining neutral to slightly positive pressure on the anterior face of the lens capsule with viscoelastic. Shallowing of the AC or drop in AC pressure results in a loss of control of the capsular tear.

Visualization of the Anterior Capsule

In cases of hypermature intumescent cataracts, it is helpful to create a small puncture in the anterior capsule, allow the cloudy liquid lens material to ooze out of the capsular bag, and aspirate this substance, clearing the view. The remainder of the capsulorhexis or "can-opener capsulotomy" can then be performed with better visualization (Gimbel and Willerscheidt 1993).

Indocyanine Green

Injecting a few drops of indocyanine green (ICG) solution onto the anterior lens capsule under air is an excellent way to stain the capsule when the red reflex is absent. Once the capsule is stained, capsulorhexis can be performed under viscoelastic. To create the ICG solution, dissolve 25 mg of ICG into

0.5 ml of the reconstitution solvent, then add 4.5 ml of BSS (Horiguchi et al. 1998).

Fiberoptic Endoilluminator (Light Pipe)

A weak or absent red reflex makes it difficult to see the anterior capsule during a capsulorhexis. A bright point light source placed at various angles near the limbus is useful for visualizing the raised edge of the capsular tear.

Instrumentation

Capsulorhexis Forceps

Capsulorhexis forceps allow excellent control of the anterior capsular flap. However, the surgeon must be able to grasp and regrasp the capsule with the jaws of the forceps, which can be quite challenging in cases with suboptimal visualization. In addition, if a sudden saccadic eye movement occurs while the capsule is in the surgeon's grasp, the rhexis can tear in an unpredictable manner, often peripheral to the pupillary border.

Bent Needle or Cystotome

One advantage of using a bent needle or cystotome is that there is no need to actually pick up the torn

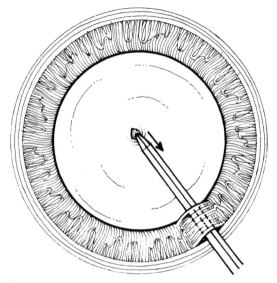

Figure 6-1. Puncture the capsule with controlled posterior pressure, keeping the forceps tips together.

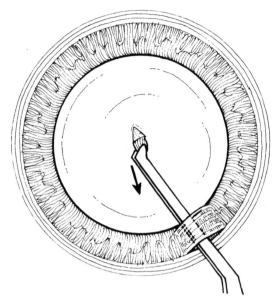

Figure 6-2. Pull the forceps toward you to create a flap.

capsular flap; pushing posteriorly on the flap near the site of the tear is all that is required. Because this technique relies solely on friction for manipulation of the capsule, however, control of the capsular tear is limited.

Capsulorhexis

A continuous-tear curvilinear capsulorhexis is preferable, although not mandatory, for phacoemulsification because of its strength and stability (Gimbel and Neuhann 1990). A capsulorhexis may be created in the following ways using a specially constructed cystotome, a bent 25-gauge or 27-gauge needle, or capsulorhexis forceps.

1. Make sure the AC is well-formed with sufficient viscoelastic. Be careful not to overinflate the AC using high-pressure injection of sodium hyaluronate, as this may drive the viscoelastic agent into the trabecular meshwork and result in postoperative IOP elevation.
2. Center the capsule in the microscope field using relatively high magnification. Focus on the anterior capsule, making sure you are not accommodating.

3. Using a bent needle, a cystotome, or the sharp tips of a capsulorhexis forceps, puncture and tear the anterior capsule to raise a free flap (Gimbel and Kaye 1997) (Figures 6-1 and 6-2). If a puncture is created without a distinct flap, grasp the edge of the punctured anterior capsule with a capsulorhexis forceps and pull it in a direction perpendicular to the edge of the capsule to create a flap.
4. Manipulate the capsular flap near the site of the tear using either friction from a bent needle or cystotome or direct grasping with a forceps.
5. Tear the capsule in a curvilinear fashion, using a slow, controlled movement (Figures 6-3 and 6-4).
6. Concentrate on directing the leading edge of the tear, being careful to prevent the tear from extending peripherally. Because there are few, if any, tactile cues in the construction of a capsulorhexis, the tear should be visualized directly at all times. In particularly difficult cases in which the cortex is milky and obscures the view of the capsular tear, viscoelastic may be required periodically to clear the view and allow positioning of the capsular flap.
7. Verify that the capsulorhexis extends for 360 degrees and that the tear connects with the origin.

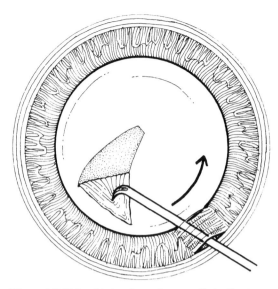

Figure 6-3. Using friction from a bent needle to direct a tear.

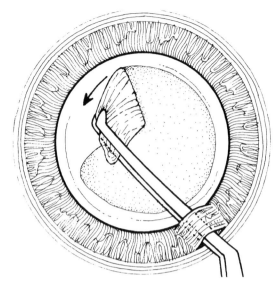

Figure 6-4. A capsulorhexis forceps provides excellent control.

If the Capsulorhexis Is Too Small

A capsulorhexis smaller than 4 mm in diameter limits access to the nucleus. The edges of a small capsulorhexis force you to maneuver the phacoemulsifier tip within a tight space, making it difficult to emulsify the nucleus in peripheral regions. With a small rhexis, the anterior capsule is often in the way of surgical maneuvers and is therefore more likely to be torn during the procedure. Furthermore, a small rhexis makes it difficult or even impossible to insert the IOL into the capsular bag.

A small rhexis is also prone to postoperative capsular phimosis, which can limit examination of the retinal periphery and may result in glare symptoms or even a loss of visual acuity if the opacified capsule encroaches on the visual axis. A Nd:YAG anterior capsulotomy should be considered in this setting to enlarge the diameter of the capsular opening. If capsular phimosis occurs across a silicone plate haptic IOL, the IOL can become deformed by the contractile forces of the capsule, inducing optical aberrations. In this situation, use the Nd:YAG laser to create a relaxing radial "incision" in the contracted anterior capsule.

In a capsulorhexis that starts out too small, the diameter of the rhexis should be increased using a spiraling technique. Rather than connect the advancing tear to the origin of the capsulorhexis,

direct the tear peripheral to the origin to create an opening of increasing diameter (Figure 6-5).

If the completed capsulorhexis is too small, create a radially oriented nick at the edge of the capsulorhexis using Vannas scissors, grasp one of the resulting flaps, and continue tearing a new, larger capsulorhexis.

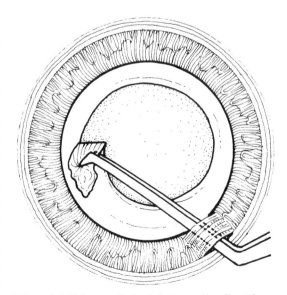

Figure 6-5. If the capsulorhexis is too small, redirect the tear into a larger spiral.

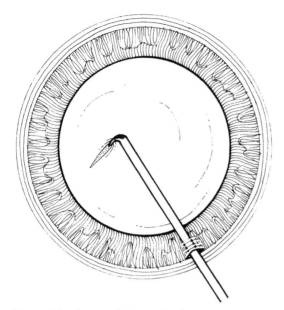

Figure 6-6. A bent needle cuts rather than tears.

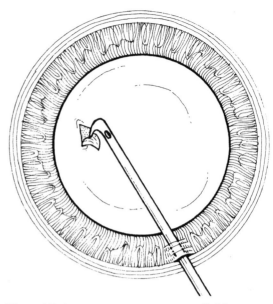

Figure 6-7. A cystotome can create a controlled flap tear.

If the Capsulorhexis Is Too Large

A capsulorhexis larger than 6 mm in diameter extends beyond the edge of most optics and may result in glare symptoms. A capsulorhexis that does not overlap the edge of the optic rarely permits optic capture by the iris in the event of AC shallowing. When tearing a large capsulorhexis, a risk of disrupting the anterior zonular insertions exists.

Can-Opener Capsulotomy

A capsulotomy is technically simpler to perform than a capsulorhexis; however, it lacks strength and structural stability. The multiple, radially oriented tears that result from a capsulotomy may extend to the zonules, the equator, and beyond under the stresses of sculpting, grooving, cracking, or chopping. Situations when conversion to a can-opener capsulotomy is indicated include an incomplete capsulorhexis or a capsulorhexis extending beneath the iris. A capsulotomy is also very useful in particularly dense cataracts in which the red reflex is absent and the anterior capsule cannot be clearly discerned. In cases with small pupils or poor visu-

alization, it is much easier to safely complete a capsulotomy than a capsulorhexis.

A cystotome, not a bent needle, is required to create a controlled capsulotomy. A cystotome has a blunt component that creates tears rather than cuts. If a bent needle is used, it creates radial cuts in the capsule (Figure 6-6) rather than the oblique tears created by a cystotome (Figure 6-7). A linear radial nick in the capsule from a sharp needle is much more likely to be propagated into the periphery than an oblique tear, which connects with neighboring tears from the cystotome.

The technique for creating a can-opener capsulotomy is as follows:

1. Insert a 27-gauge cannula into the AC and inject a volume of sodium hyaluronate sufficient to deepen the AC and maintain pupillary dilatation.
2. Withdraw the tip of the cannula as sodium hyaluronate fills the chamber to ensure even filling.
3. Place the cystotome on the anterior capsule close to the incision site.
4. Penetrate the capsule at one location and smoothly draw the cystotome centrally, creating a V-shaped tear of the capsule. The farther the length of the stroke, the longer the tear.

5. Continue in a clockwise or counterclockwise fashion, creating multiple, connecting tears (Figure 6-8).
6. Keep tears fairly close together to ensure that they all connect.

Hydrodissection

Effective phacoemulsification surgery requires free rotation of the lenticular nucleus. To achieve this degree of nuclear mobility, hydrodissection must be performed between the lens capsule and the lens cortex. Furthermore, so-called cortical-cleaving hydrodissection can obviate the need for cortical removal at the end of the surgery (Fine 1992).

Hydrodissection Technique

A round 27-gauge cannula or flat 25-gauge nucleus hydrodissector may be used in hydrodissection. A narrow (e.g., 30-gauge) cannula should only be used with caution, because the pressure from the focused stream of fluid is more likely to rupture the capsular bag. The technique for performing hydrodissection is as follows:

1. Insert the cannula tip just under the edge of the anterior capsulorhexis.
2. Advance the tip until it is approximately 2 mm distal to the edge of the capsulorhexis.
3. Angle the tip of the cannula anteriorly, tenting the anterior capsule slightly away from the cortex and establishing the appropriate cleavage plane (Figure 6-9). The position of the cannula

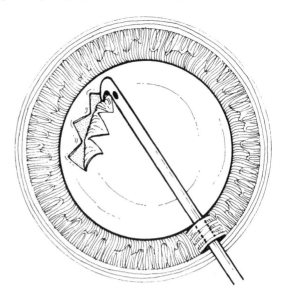

Figure 6-8. Make sure each triangular flap connects with the adjacent one.

tip before the injection of any fluid is critical; if the tip is buried even slightly in the substance of the cortex, then the cleavage plane is within the concentric lamellae of the cortex rather than between the cortex and the lenticular capsule.

4. Once the cannula tip is properly positioned, gently inject BSS while simultaneously exerting posterior pressure on the nucleus with the cannula to facilitate spreading of the fluid wave. If no posterior pressure is exerted, the BSS may not travel all the way to the opposite equatorial region, causing the portion of the lens near the cannula to prolapse anteriorly. This results in only a partial dissection.

Figure 6-9. Proper placement of the cannula tip for effective hydrodissection.

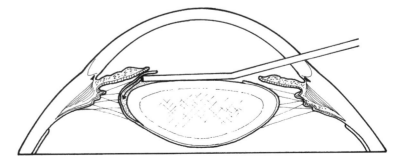

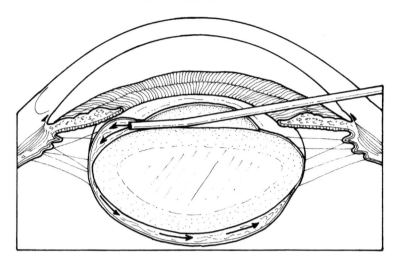

Figure 6-10. Potential posterior capsule rupture during hydrodissection owing to overinflation of the capsular bag without decompression.

5. Observe the red reflex closely as you inject BSS to watch for the advancing dissecting plane behind the nucleus. Direct visualization of this fluid wave ensures a thorough hydrodissection. If the hydrodissection cannula is not sufficiently advanced into the periphery, the BSS simply flows in a retrograde direction around the outside of the cannula and into the AC rather than advancing to dissect the corticocapsular adhesions.

Hydrodissection Learning Curve

The most common problem with hydrodissection is an inadequate dissection. If the cannula tip is not accurately positioned, no amount of fluid can disrupt the corticocapsular adhesions.

Rupturing the posterior capsule during hydrodissection is a rare but possible complication. Pushing the nucleus posteriorly after introducing each bolus of fluid helps prevent overexpansion of the capsular bag by allowing BSS to be released from the capsulorhexis edge. Failure to decompress the capsular bag may result in an expanding volume of BSS between the lens and the capsule, which can exert enough hydrostatic pressure to rupture the posterior capsule. During injection, it is critical to look for stretching of the anterior capsular rim or expansion in the circumference of the capsulorhexis, both of which are signs of an expanding capsular bag (Figure 6-10). If these signs are noted, either decompress the bag or stop injecting immediately, as a sudden posterior capsular rupture can occur in this setting.

The hydrodissection cannula can perforate the capsular bag at the equator if it is advanced too far in the periphery. It is only necessary to insert the tip of the cannula 1–2 mm peripheral to the capsulorhexis edge. The cannula should be perpendicular to the capsulorhexis edge to direct fluid peripherally and prevent fluid reflux back toward the visual axis.

If you do not achieve the proper hydrodissection plane in one location, it may be useful to move to a different area several clock hours away. Multiple partial hydrodissections can free the nucleus for rotation.

Hydrodelineation

Hydrodelineation, separating the softer concentric nuclear fibers, or epinucleus, from the more dense central fibers, may be very useful, especially when using phacoemulsification chopping techniques. Immediately after hydrodissection, the cannula may be inserted more deeply in the midperiphery of the lenticular nucleus, where the injection of BSS causes cleavage between the soft fibers of the epinuclear shell and the more dense portions of the central nucleus (Figure 6-11). When a complete hydrodelineation is performed in a case with a bright red reflex, a dramatic golden ring sign is often observed. Remember that hydrodelineation performed too centrally can result in thick outer nuclear shells, which must be removed by phacoemulsification and can prolong the procedure.

Figure 6-11. Proper placement of the cannula for hydrodelineation.

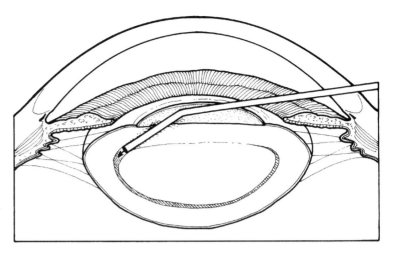

Chapter 7
Nuclear Evacuation

Rotating the Nucleus

Many techniques for nuclear evacuation rely heavily on rotating the nucleus about its anteroposterior axis. A wide range of instruments for use in nuclear rotation exists. An effective nucleus rotator should be sharp enough to engage the nucleus, yet blunt enough to avoid nuclear penetration and puncture of the capsular bag. The basic procedure is as follows:

  I. Stabilize the AC. A number of methods for creating a stable chamber exist:
     A. Aqueous/sodium hyaluronate exchange.
     B. Use of a phacoemulsifer needle. The phacoemulsifer can be set on constant irrigation. If the chamber is truly watertight, continuous infusion is not necessary.
     C. Use of an AC maintainer with an appropriate bottle height and gravity-driven inflow.
 II. Whenever possible, use a bimanual technique (generally the phacoemulsification tip and a nucleus manipulator) to counteract forces on the capsular bag and prevent zonular dehiscence.
III. Engage the nucleus with both instruments, preferably in a crevice, without pushing through to the posterior capsule.
IV. Use both instruments to rotate the nucleus either clockwise or counterclockwise, being careful to pivot the shafts of the instruments within the incisions to prevent deformation of the globe, which results in corneal striae.

Inability to Rotate the Nucleus

The most common cause of an inability to rotate the nucleus is inadequate hydrodissection. Always consider further hydrodissection if the nucleus does not rotate easily. The use of excessive force during rotational maneuvers can tear zonules and the capsule. After a properly performed hydrodissection, the nucleus should rotate easily in any direction.

Entering the Anterior Chamber with the Phacoemulsifier Tip

With the bevel down, the AC wound is easily entered, and the phacoemulsifier tip is unlikely to snag on the iris during insertion. Depending on your technique, you may need to rotate the phacoemulsifier handpiece 180 degrees for subsequent maneuvers.

With the bevel up, no need exists to rotate the tip for most maneuvers, but the tip tends to drag and distort the lip of the incision, and the posterior portion of the bevel can become snagged in the iris with even minimal AC shallowing.

Equipment Settings

Phacoemulsifier Power

The phacoemulsifier power determines the amplitude of the ultrasonic vibration and therefore the energy of each cycle. Use the lowest power setting that still emulsifies the nucleus easily. If the power is too low, the nucleus is not emulsified and cannot be aspirated into the phacoemulsifier tip; if the power is too high, excessive energy is imparted to the corneal endothelium, and there is potential for an incision burn.

Phacoemulsifier Pulse

Some phacoemulsifiers offer a "pulse mode" in which power is pulsed on and off intermittently. This setting is helpful for emulsifying and aspirating free nuclear fragments in a controlled fashion.

Vacuum Level

A high vacuum level allows the phacoemulsifier tip to firmly hold the nucleus during chopping maneuvers, provided the lumen is completely occluded. When emulsifying free nuclear fragments, use high vacuum levels to keep the fragments at the tip as they are emulsified and aspirated. Sudden release of the luminal occlusion in the presence of a high vacuum level can produce a surge effect. If this occurs during the emulsification and aspiration of a nuclear fragment, the chamber may abruptly collapse, causing the posterior capsule to strike the phacoemulsifier tip. Alternatively, if the occlusion is released as the phacoemulsifier tip emulsifies through the nucleus in the periphery, the resulting surge can cause either the iris or the posterior capsule to enter the tip. The surge effect can be reduced by using an aspiration bypass tip (Aspiration Bypass System, Alcon, Ft. Worth, TX).

When performing sculpting maneuvers, little or no vacuum is needed to prevent the nucleus from being pulled toward the phacoemulsifier tip, potentially stressing the zonules.

Aspiration Flow Rate

Aspiration flow rate is proportional to the speed at which nuclear fragments approach the phacoemulsifier tip. Other than a slower progression of the surgery, no disadvantage exists to a low-flow rate. Higher flow rates allow phacoemulsification to pro-

ceed at a faster pace and therefore permit the posterior capsule to enter the phacoemulsifier tip quickly.

Infusion Bottle Height

The height of the infusion bottle determines the hydrostatic pressure of the irrigating solution. If a true closed system is maintained during the surgery, the bottle height may be quite low. If leakage occurs around the phacoemulsifier tip or at a paracentesis site, the bottle height may need to be increased to maintain a deep chamber. The bottle may also need to be raised if there is positive vitreous pressure.

Sculpting

Sculpting the nucleus is a very useful skill to master. When sculpting, use a 30- or 45-degree tip. A zero- or 15-degree tip is easily occluded, leading to unwanted aspiration of the lens. Be sure the tip is never completely occluded and use a low vacuum setting. Allow the needle to advance as the resistance in front of the tip is emulsified. When done properly, sculpting shaves off layers of the nucleus with exquisite control without subjecting the capsular bag or zonules to any undesirable forces. It is easier to judge depth in the nuclear periphery rather than in the center, where the angle of the tip is much steeper. Nonetheless, deep central sculpting is critical to the success of this technique. Be sure to account for the anatomic curve of the posterior lens surface when making long sculpting passes.

Inexperienced surgeons are often faced with the problem of not knowing how close the phacoemulsifier tip is to the posterior capsule. With a dense PSC plaque, it is often possible to maintain a view of the posterior capsule quite clearly. In many cases, however, no distinct visual cues exist to guide the surgeon. Experience and knowing that the anteroposterior diameter of the lenticular nucleus is usually four to five tip widths help guide the surgeon. When phacoemulsifying particularly brunescent cataracts, the intensity of the red reflex is an indicator of how much lens nucleus remains between the phacoemulsifier tip and the posterior capsule. The brown or white color at the center of the nucleus becomes more translucent as the red reflex appears more posteriorly. In addition, owing to regional differences in lens density, the central nucleus typically requires greater power than the peripheral areas just anterior to the posterior capsule. Periodically, the surgeon may wish to pause to readjust the fine focus on the microscope to maintain a sharp view of the central nuclear lamellae. If the surgeon is not comfortable with the depth of the phacoemulsifier needle, the tip may be withdrawn from the eye and viscoelastic may be injected to clear away nuclear debris and enhance the quality of the stereoscopic view.

One-Handed Technique

Although the phacoemulsifier tip's primary function is to emulsify and aspirate the lenticular nucleus, it can also be used as a manipulating instrument to facilitate nuclear removal. The following steps describe the one-handed technique of nuclear extraction:

1. Center the eye in the microscope field, using appropriate focus and magnification.

2. Introduce the ultrasonic tip into the AC.

3. Sculpt the central nucleus until a thin central layer remains (Figure 7-1). Advance the tip at the same rate as the nucleus is emulsified, gliding through the lens material rather than dragging or pushing the lens. Advancing the handpiece too quickly pushes the lens and capsule away from you, stressing on the zonules in the meridian of the incision.

4. To spin the nucleus, engage the peripheral nuclear shelf with a portion of the bevel. Discontinue phacoemulsification, aspiration, and irrigation and allow the chamber to shallow. Rotate the nucleus by nudging the peripheral shelf.

5. Continue to sculpt and remove the central nucleus, rotating it as necessary to access various regions of the lens. Concentrate on shaving the nucleus rather than emulsifying through it. If the phacoemulsifier tip advances past the peripheral nucleus, you may rupture the posterior capsule (Figure 7-2). Furthermore, if you perforate the nuclear shell, the nucleus becomes impaled on the tip and must be pushed away with a second instrument (Figure 7-3).

6. When the central nucleus has been shaved to a thin plate, the nuclear bowl begins to collapse inward as emulsification proceeds in the periphery.

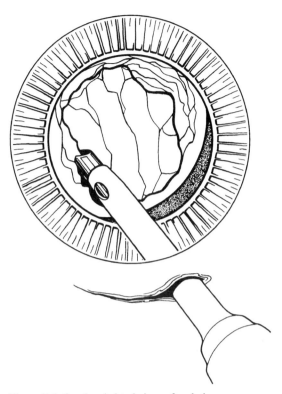

Figure 7-1. One-handed technique of sculpting.

At this point, occlude the tip and use aspiration to draw the periphery toward the center, which encourages collapse of the nuclear bowl. Once the nuclear shell collapses centrally, ultrasound power can be used to emulsify and aspirate the remaining nucleus. In some cases, it may be necessary to allow the AC to collapse to mobilize the posterior plate.

Nucleus Cracking

Nucleus cracking with the use of a specially designed cracker is a very straightforward and fairly simple technique to master and includes the following steps:

1. Create a groove in the central nucleus using the phacoemulsifier tip. The groove should be slightly wider than the tip to accommodate the irrigation sleeve, but its walls should be as vertical as possible to maximize contact area between the cracker blades and the nucleus. The groove need only be as long as the cracker blades, but should be

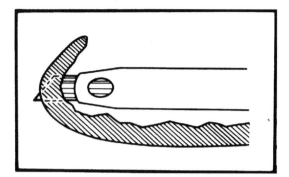

Figure 7-2. Avoid advancing the phacoemulsifier tip *through* the nucleus when sculpting.

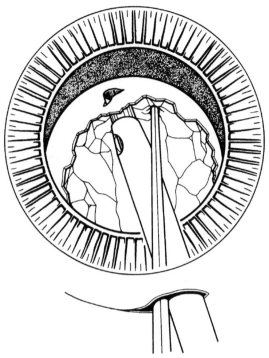

Figure 7-3. Use a second instrument to push away the impaled nuclear shell.

at least three-fourths of the depth of the central nucleus to achieve a complete crack extending all the way to the posterior cortex (Figure 7-4).

2. If a cracker is used, inject viscoelastic into the AC overlying the groove to maintain chamber depth during the cracking maneuver. If cracking is performed using the phacoemulsifier tip and a second instrument, constant irrigation can be used during the maneuver.

3. Rotate the nucleus 90 degrees with a second instrument and sculpt a second groove perpendicular to the first, thereby bisecting one of the heminuclei. Again, create this groove with adequate depth and vertical walls.

4. Again use the cracker to split the heminucleus into two quadrants.

5. Rotate the nucleus 180 degrees and repeat the procedure for the other heminucleus.

6. After creating four distinct quadrants, phacoemulsify each one, using aspiration to draw the quadrants away from the capsular bag (Gimbel 1991).

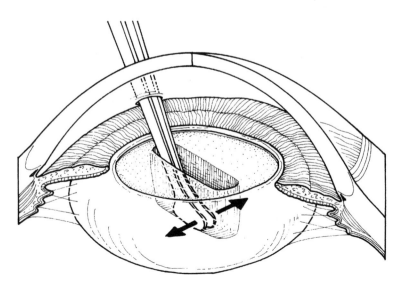

Figure 7-4. A nucleus cracker placed deep inside the trough. Note the vertical walls of the trough.

Bimanual Technique

Although the phacoemulsifier tip can be used as a manipulating instrument in addition to emulsifying and aspirating the nucleus, having a second instrument in the eye often facilitates maneuvers.

Bimanual nuclear evacuation has several advantages over the one-handed technique. Using two instruments simultaneously through two ports greatly enhances the stability of the eye in surgeries performed using topical anesthesia. Separating the two instruments by an angle of 90 degrees maximizes control, as the globe cannot rotate about any axis with the instruments so placed. Furthermore, the use of two instruments allows numerous techniques for mechanical fragmentation of the nucleus without the use of ultrasound power, thereby reducing the amount of ultrasound energy delivered to the iris and corneal endothelium.

Second Instruments

Second instruments are available in a variety of shapes and sizes. Although no single best second instrument exists, certain manipulators are preferable for particular techniques. In general, second instruments should have blunt tips to protect the posterior capsule. Chopping instruments may have an edge, although this is certainly not required. Instruments used to rotate the nucleus should be sharp enough to engage the nucleus for optimum control, yet blunt enough to prevent capsular rupture.

"Crack and Flip"

In the "crack and flip" technique, hydrodelineation is performed, then the nucleus is grooved and cracked into four quadrants using the phacoemulsifier tip and a second instrument. Once the quadrants are removed, the remaining epinucleus is trimmed and flipped over to facilitate its removal (Fine et al. 1993).

"Chip and Flip"

In the "chip and flip" technique, a nuclear bowl is first created using the one-handed technique. Depending on your experience, a second instrument is used to facilitate nuclear rotation while you emulsify the entire rim of the nuclear bowl. Engage the remaining nuclear chip using vacuum with the phacoemulsifier tip and assistance from the second instrument. Once the dense posterior nucleus is emulsified and aspirated, slide the remaining epinuclear shell away from the incision, completely inverting it. Use phacoemulsification to emulsify the remaining epinucleus (Fine 1991).

Nucleus Chopping

Chopping requires greater skill and practice than cracking; however, it affords the additional advantage of segmenting the nucleus quickly and with minimal ultrasound energy. Controversy exists over whether irrigation or ultrasound energy has the most significant effect on the corneal endothelium. In a "phaco-chop," the nucleus is held stationary using high vacuum from the phacoemulsifier tip while the chopper mechanically fragments the nucleus (Nagahara 1993a, b). It is critical to use a fairly high vacuum and completely occlude the phacoemulsifier tip with nuclear material to stabilize the nucleus effectively. Keeping the foot pedal in a position, using irrigation-aspiration without ultrasound, stabilizes the nucleus. Changing to phacoemulsification dislodges the nucleus from the phacoemulsifier tip and makes the chopping maneuver very difficult to perform.

1. Enter the nucleus with the phacoemulsifier tip using a quick burst of power and then use aspiration only to stabilize the nucleus.
2. Carefully place the chopper posterior to the lip of the anterior capsule and slide it peripherally, remaining parallel to the anterior surface of the nucleus within the anterior cortex (Figure 7-5A).
3. As you reach the periphery of the central nucleus, rotate the chopper so that the tip is pointing posteriorly towards the posterior capsule (Figure 7-5A, B).
4. Draw the chopper centrally, toward the phacoemulsifier tip, in a smooth and controlled fashion, transecting the nucleus (Figures 7-6 and 7-7).

This maneuver may be repeated multiple times to divide the nucleus in half and then into smaller

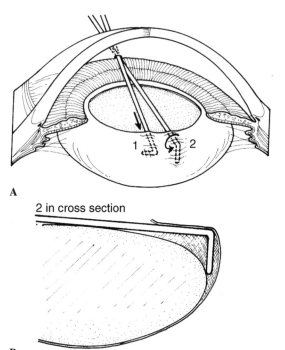

A

2 in cross section

B

Figure 7-5. A. A chopper is placed just posterior to the anterior capsule (1). Once past the lens equator, the chopper is rotated into a vertical orientation (2). **B.** Proper positioning of the chopper just before initiating a chopping maneuver.

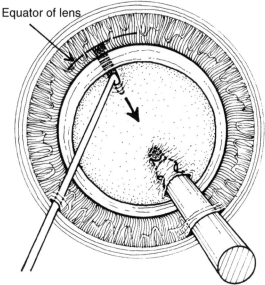

Equator of lens

Figure 7-6. Chopping the nucleus in half without creating a central groove.

fragments (Figure 7-8). A vacuum level of at least 100 mm Hg should be used to stabilize the nucleus on the phacoemulsifier tip. Be aware that surge or collapse of the AC may result from the use of high vacuum settings; using an ABS (Aspiration Bypass System, Alcon, Ft. Worth, TX) micro tip for the phacoemulsification handpiece and high-vacuum tubing with a small internal diameter and large exterior walls may reduce the incidence of surge.

Several other methods of nuclear fragmentation exist, including combinations of cracking and chop-

ping, such as "stop and chop" phacoemulsification (Koch and Katzen 1994).

"Quick Chop"

When using chopping techniques, placement of the chopper in the periphery at the lens equator often proves difficult. The use of the "quick chop" technique avoids this maneuver altogether. In a quick chop, the chopper tip is placed on the anterior surface of the nucleus, well within the boundaries of the capsulorhexis. The nucleus is engaged with the phacoemulsifier tip using high vacuum, and the chopper is pushed posteriorly while the tip is pulled anteriorly (Figure 7-9). This creates a chop in the

Figure 7-7. Proper placement of the chopper in the periphery, just before a chopping maneuver. Note that the phacoemulsifier tip is deep within the nucleus.

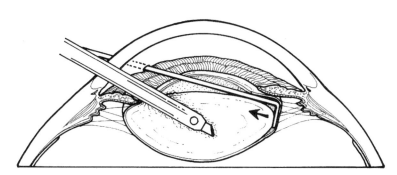

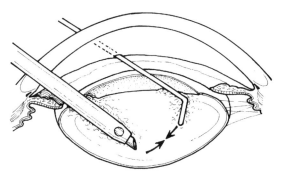

Figure 7-9. Push the chopper into the nucleus and pull toward the phacoemulsifier tip to fragment the nucleus.

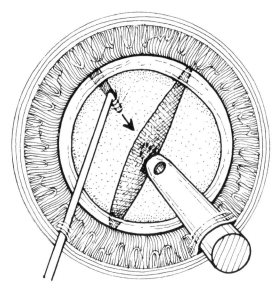

Figure 7-8. Use a chopping maneuver to free a wedge.

lens that can be propagated by moving the two instruments laterally in opposite directions (Vasavada 1996). This technique offers tremendous advantages in small-pupil cases, when safe placement of the chopping instrument in the periphery is nearly impossible.

Nuclear "Prechopping"

The technique of nuclear "prechopping" (Akahoshi 1996) fragments the nucleus mechanically rather than using ultrasound energy.

Two identical phacoemulsifier choppers are used. Each instrument should be at least 2 mm long at its distal 90-degree bend. The tips of the choppers must be rounded and finely polished to prevent trauma to the lens capsule.

Hydrodissection and hydrodelineation are critical for this procedure, and should be performed as described in Chapter 6.

When learning nuclear prechopping, begin by aspirating anterior lens cortex using the phacoemulsification handpiece without ultrasound. Keep the phacoemulsifier tip in a bevel-down position and sweep it in a circular motion within the capsular opening to remove as much anterior cortex as possible. Removing this cortical material allows better visualization of the lens, and less cor-

tical debris is loosened during the chopping maneuvers. Initially, performing the chopping maneuvers under viscoelastic is very useful until you become more facile with the technique.

Place the two choppers at the nuclear equator, 90 degrees apart. Insert the instruments nearly parallel to the iris, between the anterior capsule and the anterior surface of the central nucleus. Rotate each chopper so that the blunt end faces the posterior capsule at the equatorial region of the lens.

In a smooth, controlled motion, paying careful attention to the lens and capsule anatomy, pull the choppers together toward the visual axis while exerting slight posterior pressure (Figure 7-10A) to prevent the choppers from skating over the anterior surface of the nucleus. The lens is thus mechanically chopped in half. Fragment one heminucleus into quadrants using a similar technique (Figure 7-10B). Rotate the lens fragments 180 degrees and bisect the remaining heminucleus using the same chopping maneuver (Figure 7-10C).

Because it minimizes trauma from ultrasound energy and irrigation-aspiration, nuclear prechopping is well suited for elderly patients with compromised endothelial function, patients with Fuchs' endothelial dystrophy, and patients with corneal grafts. Furthermore, the direction of the forces applied in this technique places minimal stress on the lens capsule and zonules, making the procedure useful in cases of pseudoexfoliation, phacodonesis, and lens subluxation.

However, nuclear prechopping requires considerable practice and bimanual dexterity. It relies on fine motor control and mastery of the spatial relationships in the anterior segment. The most significant risk of this procedure is the potential placement

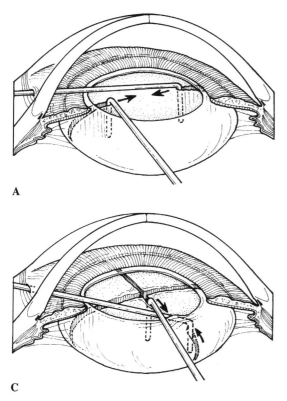

A

B

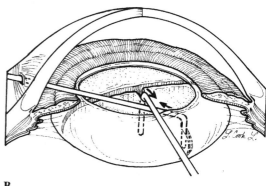

Figure 7-10. A. Pull the two choppers together, keeping their tips deep within the nucleus. **B.** Bisect the heminucleus by placing one chopper in the newly formed crack. **C.** Bisect the remaining heminucleus after rotating the lens fragments 180 degrees.

C

of the choppers in the sulcus outside the lens capsule, which can result in rupturing of the zonules and disinsertion of the capsular bag.

Supracapsular Phacoemulsification

To execute supracapsular phacoemulsification, a large (6 mm or larger) capsulorhexis is created, and a very thorough hydrodissection is performed. Posterior pressure is then exerted in the periphery to flip the lenticular nucleus within the capsular bag, bringing the posterior surface of the nucleus anteriorly and the entire lens anterior to the anterior capsule (Maloney and Dillman 1997). Because the posterior surface of the nucleus has a smaller radius of curvature than the anterior surface, the inverted lens allows easier access to the phacoemulsifier tip and a variety of one-handed or two-handed techniques is possible. Supracapsular phacoemulsification purportedly allows higher aspiration flow rates, which may increase the efficiency of emulsification (Maloney and Dillman 1997).

Some surgeons advocate placing the lens entirely in the AC. Although this may protect the posterior capsule during phacoemulsification, it puts the corneal endothelium at risk by placing it closer to the vibrating ultrasound tip and also leaves the cornea exposed to any freely circulating nuclear fragments.

Planned Extracapsular Nucleus Expression

With advanced phacoemulsification techniques, it is rarely necessary to perform a planned extracapsular nuclear expression. However, it is occasionally useful to convert a phacoemulsification case to a nuclear-expression technique.

Conversion from Phacoemulsification to Nuclear Expression

When first learning phacoemulsification, you should have a low threshold for conversion to nuclear expression. Indications for conversion include (1) poor visualization, (2) repeated iris trauma with the phacoemulsifier tip, (3) a small pupil, and (4) a technical malfunction in the phacoemulsification unit.

Other possible indications for conversion include

1. If, during phacoemulsification, posterior capsular rupture or vitreous prolapse into the AC occurs and a significant portion of the nucleus remains.
2. If the nucleus is so firm that 100% phacoemulsifier power is inadequate for emulsification (this is extremely rare).

Numerous techniques for converting to extracapsular cataract expression exist. The following is a straightforward procedure that yields consistent results.

1. Perform a sodium hyaluronate/aqueous exchange to stabilize the AC.
2. Enlarge the capsulorhexis, if necessary, or create a can-opener capsulotomy.
3. Enlarge your incision in the manner in which it was created. For a scleral tunnel incision, extend the initial scleral groove and continue the plane of the lamellar scleral dissection. In a clear cornea case, the corneal wound may be carefully enlarged in the proper plane, but you should bear in mind the possible need for sutures at the end of the surgery, which may result in postoperative astigmatism. Alternatively, a corneal wound may be left to self-seal, and a longer scleral tunnel incision may be made in a new location.

Regardless of its architecture, the incision should be large enough to permit smooth delivery of the remaining nucleus. Bear in mind that lens nuclei vary in size and each patient must be considered individually. Note that the chord length of the incision must not only be long enough to accommodate the linear size of the remaining nucleus, but wide enough to accommodate the thickness of the central lens. For the beginner, incision size is a particularly important detail. During expression of the lens through a tight incision, numerous complications may arise, including tumbling of the nucleus, endothelial cell loss, rupture of zonules, and vitreous loss.

4. Using a muscle hook, gently apply superiorly directed pressure at the inferior limbus while pulling the iris toward you with an iris retractor and

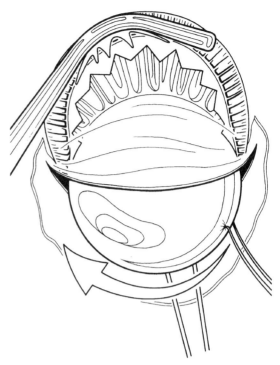

Figure 7-11. Rotating the nucleus during extracapsular expression.

applying posterior pressure to the posterior lip of the incision.

5. Do not slide the muscle hook across the cornea; this may result in lens-endothelial contact, which can lead to endothelial compromise.

6. Have an assistant extract the nucleus by using a bent 25-gauge needle to rotate it about its antero-posterior axis while pulling it out of the incision (Figure 7-11). If no assistant is available, release the muscle hook once the superior portion of the nucleus begins to prolapse though the incision and use the bent 25-gauge needle in the manner described previously.

7. Once the nucleus presents through the incision, immediately release pressure on the globe to prevent the mechanical prolapse of vitreous.

8. Once the nucleus is removed from the eye, reapproximate the wound edges as quickly as possible to decrease the risk of a choroidal hemorrhage. Preplaced sutures clearly offer an advantage in this regard; however, considerable time and attention is required with preplaced sutures to create suture loops that neither entrap the prolapsing nucleus nor slip free from the tissue.

9. When reapproximating the wound edges, leave a residual opening wide enough to accommodate the optic of the lens implant. This can be accomplished with either an interrupted or a running suture.

10. The remaining incision opening may require temporary interrupted suture(s) to create a closed system for effective irrigation-aspiration cortical cleanup.

11. Use automated irrigation-aspiration to remove residual cortical material, using either the bimanual or one-handed technique.

12. Use a capsule polisher to loosen any cortical debris in the visual axis and to remove any residual adherent lens epithelial cells, which may lead to capsular opacification.

13. Inject viscoelastic to inflate the capsular bag, and place the lens implant within the bag using a lens inserter or Kelman-McPherson forceps. First, place the distal loop into the bag, followed by the optic and finally the trailing loop. Place the latter using a Kelman-McPherson forceps with posterior pressure applied with a Sinskey hook.

14. Use irrigation-aspiration again to remove residual viscoelastic material.

15. Reapproximate the remaining wound opening using additional 10-0 nylon interrupted sutures.

16. Apply gentle pressure on the globe using A-cellulose spear cell sponges to confirm watertight closure.

17. Reapproximate the conjunctiva either with interrupted 10-0 nylon sutures (being careful to bury the knots subconjunctivally) or with bipolar cautery. Bipolar cautery is often quicker, but may result in scarring of the conjunctiva and irregularities on the conjunctival surface that can lead to excess lacrimation or foreign-body sensation. Excessive manipulation and scarring of the conjunctiva may negatively affect any future glaucoma surgeries.

18. Remove the wire-lid speculum, taking care not to disturb the reapproximated conjunctival incision.

Intracapsular Cataract Extraction

With the high success rate of extracapsular cataract surgery, few if any indications for intracapsular cataract extraction exist, although a variety of intracapsular techniques have been described (Osher 1975; Jaffe 1972).

Chapter 8
Removal of Cortex

Although technically challenging, cortical cleaving hydrodissection, if performed skillfully, frees the cortex and allows most of it to be aspirated during phacoemulsification (Fine 1992). Nonetheless, irrigation-aspiration to remove residual cortical material is usually required after nuclear extraction.

A number of techniques exist for removing residual cortical material from the lens capsule. The simplest requires only a syringe and a blunt cannula; however, this method is tedious and can cause AC collapse.

Automated irrigation-aspiration is a safe, controlled method of cortical removal and can be performed using either the one-handed or bimanual technique.

When using a one-handed combined irrigation-aspiration probe, subincisional cortex can be difficult to access. Many capsular tears in phacoemulsification cases are actually caused by automated irrigation-aspiration, particularly at subincisional locations. Use a curved irrigation-aspiration cannula to facilitate removal of subincisional cortex (Figure 8-1).

An alternative technique is a bimanual system (Katena Products, Inc., Denville, NJ), in which 21-gauge irrigation-aspiration cannulas are placed through separate 0.5-mm ports. These cannulas are used interchangeably through both ports, accessing cortex from opposite sides of the capsular bag (Figure 8-2) and eliminating the difficulties associated with subincisional cortex. An added advantage of the bimanual technique is that the irrigation cannula can be used to mechanically disrupt dense cortical

or residual epinuclear material, which can clog the aspiration port.

An AC maintainer may also be used for cortical removal. This allows the use of a more streamlined aspiration cannula inserted through a separate side port, but subincisional cortex may be difficult to access unless the aspiration cannula and AC maintainer are exchanged, as in the bimanual technique.

Automated Cortical Removal

The following steps are used in automated removal of cortical material:

1. Using irrigation only, place the aspirating port (facing anteriorly) in the periphery, just posterior to the plane of targeted cortex.
2. Use low vacuum to grasp the free edge of the cortical sheet.
3. Increase the vacuum while pulling the cannula toward the visual axis, using a combination of aspiration and mechanical pulling to peel sheets of cortex away from the capsular fornix and posterior capsule (Figures 8-3 and 8-4).

Constant vigilance is required during aspiration of cortical material, as the posterior capsule can quickly occlude the aspiration port, causing an opening in the capsule. Avoid directing the aspirating port posteriorly; the posterior capsule can be engaged in a fraction of a second (Figure 8-5A). With the port

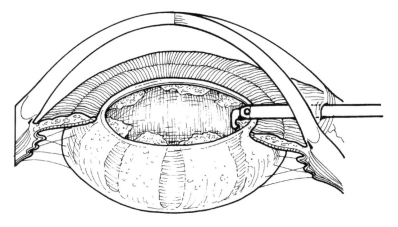

Figure 8-1. An angled irrigation-aspiration tip easily engages subincisional cortex.

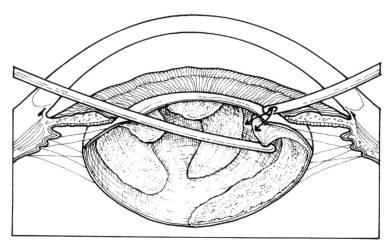

Figure 8-2. Bimanual technique eliminates difficulty with subincisional cortex.

facing anteriorly, it is possible to aspirate the iris or even the posterior capsule in the periphery (Figure 8-5B), owing to the anteriorly sloping angle of the posterior capsule near the equatorial region.

Residual cortical material that proves difficult to remove (particularly subincisional cortex) should be left in place. Leaving a small amount of residual cortex is preferable to creating an opening in the posterior capsule and marring an otherwise flawless surgery.

Removal of Anterior Capsular Tags

If a continuous circular capsulorhexis is not created, tags, or flaps of AC, may remain as a result. Occasionally, these can affect the pupillary border and even the optical clarity of the visual axis.

Depending on their location and size, these tags may be trimmed with Vannas scissors. Alternatively, the following technique may be useful:

1. Position the irrigation-aspiration probe directly posterior to the isthmus of the flap.
2. Aspirate this portion of the flap into the port using high vacuum.
3. Using a Sinskey hook or a bent needle, perforate the capsule overlying the irrigation-aspiration port to create a nidus for a capsular tear.
4. Use high vacuum to tear away the tag and draw the capsular remnant into the port.
5. If the free capsular fragment becomes lodged at the port and cannot be aspirated, simply withdraw the cannula out of the AC along with the adherent capsular fragment.

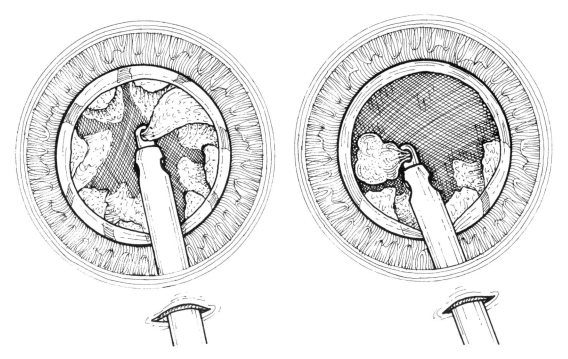

Figure 8-3. Engaging and stripping cortex.

Figure 8-4. Once cortex is "grasped" by the aspiration port, strip cortex from the capsule by pulling centrally.

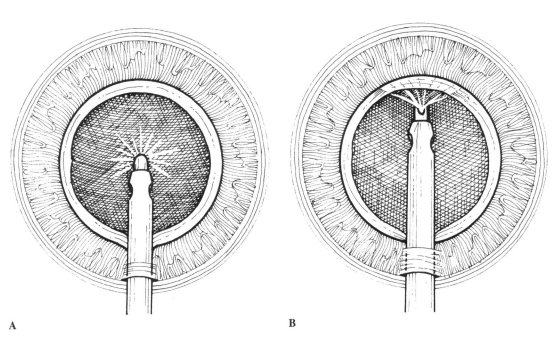

A

B

Figure 8-5. A. Avoid using irrigation-aspiration with the port facing the posterior capsule. **B.** Even an anteriorly facing port can engage posterior capsule in the periphery.

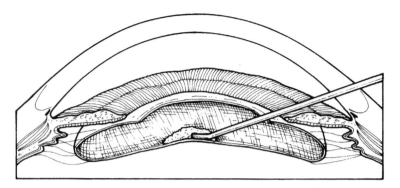

Figure 8-6. Polishing residual cortical material with the posterior capsule in a convex configuration.

Polishing the Posterior Capsule

Before inserting the lens implant, ensure that the visual axis is optically clear. Polishing capsules that appear to be optically transparent may be beneficial, as clear cortical layers invisible to the surgeon may be present. Furthermore, epithelial cell migration from the equatorial lens capsule to the posterior capsule can occur before surgery. These epithelial cells, if left in place on the posterior capsule, may result in rapid formation of Elschnig pearls or fibrosis postoperatively.

To polish the capsule safely:

1. Keep the AC slightly shallow to put the posterior capsule in a convex position (Figure 8-6). If the posterior capsule is concave, the capsule polisher must be at a very steep angle to access the cortical debris, which increases the risk of capsular perforation. Furthermore, with a concave posterior capsule, no countertraction on the capsule exists and tears can occur more readily.

2. Using a circular or back-and-forth motion, gently remove cellular debris, especially clear linear strands of cortex on the posterior capsule, with a carbide-impregnated tip such as a 23-gauge irrigating Kratz capsule scraper (see Figure 8-6). Alternatively, use a silicone Terry Squeegee (Alcon Surgical Inc., Fort Worth, TX).

3. Keep the posterior capsule taut, as wrinkles in the capsule may snag on the polishing instrument, causing a tear.

Chapter 9
Intraocular Lens

Enlarging the Wound

With few exceptions, an IOL requires a larger incision than a phacoemulsification needle. Some lens delivery systems for foldable IOLs allow insertion through nonenlarged wounds, although these systems can result in increased wound size secondary to stretching.

The wound should be enlarged enough for the IOL to be placed through the incision without undue force. Forcing an IOL through an incision that is too small may cause irregular tearing of the wound edges or distortion of the wound margins, which can result in loss of a watertight seal or induced astigmatism. Use of excessive force with a tight incision may also result in sudden entry into the AC, resulting in posterior capsular rupture, zonular dehiscence, or trauma to the iris or corneal endothelium.

When enlarging a corneal incision, it is best to cut only when entering the AC and not when exiting; this helps ensure a smooth incision with an adequate internal length. Concentrate on enlarging the wound in the original plane in a smooth, linear fashion, using a sharp crescent blade or appropriately sized keratome.

When enlarging a triplanar corneal scleral tunnel, reproduce all three planes along the entire length of the enlarged incision. Enlarge the wound with the same care and precision used to construct the original incision. Although it may be tempting to simply use a sawing motion at one end of the incision, this jeopardizes the self-sealing properties of the initial wound.

Selecting an Intraocular Lens

Over the years, myriad IOL innovations and designs have emerged. The ideal IOL satisfies the following requirements (Bahadur and Sinskey 1998):

- Complete biocompatibility
- Resistance to bacterial adherence
- Easy intraoperative insertion
- Excellent centration and stability
- High refractive index
- Optical properties maximizing visual function without distortion or glare
- Ease of removal (if necessary)

Although an IOL's primary function is achieving a desired refractive result, it also contributes to intraocular stability and should be used even if the intended correction entails a zero-power IOL (Kohnen et al. 1996).

Spheric-power IOLs placed parallel to the iris plane do not induce any cylindrical power. An IOL that tilts results in plus cylinder at the axis of optic rotation. Tilted IOLs are quite rare, but may be seen in certain circumstances, such as scleral fixation of an IOL placed in the ciliary sulcus or an AC IOL too small for an eye. Less commonly, capsular contraction and fibrosis can play a role in optic tilt and even deformation of the optic's curvature, especially with the use of silicone plate haptic IOLs or those with polypropylene loops.

Foldable Lenses

The principal advantage of a foldable lens is that it requires a shorter incision length, decreasing potential astigmatic effects and wound healing time. In our clinical experience, we have found acrylic and silicone foldable lenses to be comparable in their properties, although some debate exists as to the degree of inflammation induced by each. Acrylic lenses appear to result in less glare and more contrast sensitivity than their silicone counterparts (Kohnen et al. 1996). Silicone lenses require extra practice and care when performing a Nd:YAG laser capsulotomy in cases of postoperative posterior chamber opacification.

Loop Haptics and Plate Haptics

Over the years, ophthalmologists have become imprecise in their references to nonoptic portions of the lens. Technically, the nonoptic portion should be called a *haptic*. There are plate haptics and loop haptics, among others. Loop haptics may be termed *loops*, but should not be referred to merely as haptics, as this is imprecise and potentially misleading.

Loop haptics are preferable to plate haptics for a number of reasons. Plate haptic IOLs are fixed in size and thus cannot conform to the shape or size of the capsular bag. In fact, fibrosis of the lens capsule can actually bend a plate haptic IOL, distorting the optical portion and resulting in astigmatic effects or even lens dislocation (Schneiderman 1997). In a worst-case scenario, a plate haptic IOL distorted by the contractual scarring forces of the capsular bag can store potential mechanical energy that is subsequently released during Nd:YAG laser capsulotomy, propelling the IOL into the vitreous cavity. Furthermore, due to the fusion of the anterior and posterior capsules, which occurs at the holes of the haptics, these lenses are much more difficult to remove from the eye in the event of endophthalmitis, IOL power errors, decentration, or trauma.

Loop Designs

An IOL should not only be well-fitted to the patient's eye, but easily implantable as well. Loop configuration significantly impacts an IOL's ease of implantation and removal. Many surgeons think that modified J-loops are easier to manipulate than C-loops. Ease of handling is important not only for atraumatic insertion of the IOL, but for situations in which the IOL must be explanted. Some surgeons point out that Miyake views of lens capsules containing IOLs demonstrate that C-loops have a broader arc of contact with the equatorial region of the capsular bag, and therefore distribute forces more evenly than J- or modified J-loops. Whether this arc of contact is of any clinical significance is controversial.

Loop Angulation

When the first posterior-chamber IOLs with no loop angulation were positioned in the ciliary sulcus, the optic was very close to the posterior surface of the iris and could cause pupillary block or pupillary capture of the IOL. In the past, loops were angulated to create a small gap between the pupillary plane and the anterior surface of the optic, thus preventing pupillary capture. Now that most IOLs are placed inside the capsular bag and cataract wounds are self-sealing with stable postoperative ACs, loop angulation is no longer necessary to prevent IOL capture. In fact, posterior displacement of the IOL relative to the entrance pupil actually promotes edge glare. Light rays entering a 5-mm pupil from the far periphery, for example, strike the opposite edge of a well-centered 5.5-mm optic if the optic is significantly posterior to the iris plane (Figures 9-1 and 9-2).

Three-Piece Lenses

Three-piece IOLs are inherently more flexible than their one-piece counterparts. Added flexibility results in smooth, controlled motions during implantation and, if necessary, during removal. Struggling with the implantation or explantation of a rigid IOL can result in trauma to the intraoperative capsular bag, corneal endothelium, and iris.

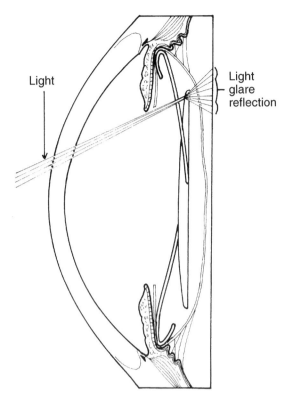

Figure 9-1. A posteriorly vaulted optic allows edge glare even with central light rays.

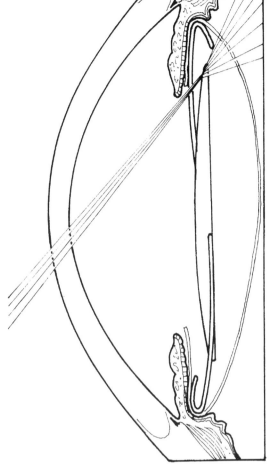

Figure 9-2. Minimal loop angulation results in glare only from the far periphery.

Multifocal Lenses

As of this writing, multifocal IOLs appear to be a promising avenue (Vaquero et al. 1996). Newer refractive designs have clear advantages over their diffractive counterparts (Pieh et al. 1998). Although some patients with multifocal IOLs are quite pleased with the quality of their near and distant vision, a significant number of patients still requires glasses for certain tasks that rely on near or distant vision. For optimum results, multifocal IOLs should be implanted bilaterally.

Careful patient selection is critical when considering a multifocal lens. Patients who are very aware of subtle visual changes, those with occupations or hobbies requiring sharp vision without distortions or halos, and those with macular pathology should carefully weigh the relative advantages of multifocal versus unifocal IOLs.

Toric Lenses

Toric IOLs appear to provide a reasonable option for the correction of astigmatism at the time of cataract surgery. Toric IOLs can eliminate the need for corneal refractive incisions, which can permanently weaken the globe and introduce risks of perforation or infection. On the other hand, toric IOLs must be placed with great precision and must not rotate significantly in the postoperative period for their effect to be preserved (Shimizu et al. 1994). Further studies and long-term follow-up are required to better evaluate the efficacy of these lens implants.

Hydrogel Lenses

Hydrogel lenses demonstrate excellent biocompatibility and are resistant to Nd:YAG laser damage. However, these lenses may be more adherent to pigment cells than polymethylmethacrylate (PMMA) IOLs (Chehade and Elder 1997). Some hydrogel IOL designs include PMMA loop haptics seamlessly bonded onto the hydrogel haptic, combining the advantages of a foldable lens with those of a one-piece IOL.

Characteristics of the Lens Implant

Materials

Biocompatibility is perhaps the most important characteristic of an IOL. PMMA, with its long history of biological inertness, is clearly the gold standard for IOL materials. With modern-day small incision cataract surgery, however, a foldable material is necessary. Acrylic and silicone are the most popular of these.

Insertion systems for silicone lenses have been developed that permit precise, controlled IOL implantation through a small incision. Nonetheless, these delivery systems have not eliminated the problems associated with silicone itself, such as its tenacious adherence to silicone oil during retinal surgery (Apple et al. 1996). Furthermore, silicone may result in increased fibrosis of the posterior capsule (Oshika et al. 1998; Mamalis et al. 1996) and decreased contrast sensitivity (Johansen et al. 1997).

Acrylic IOLs, on the other hand, are compatible with silicone oil surgery and, in our experience, have been well tolerated. Acrylic does have a tendency to stick to itself and to the inserter in the operating room, but this is easily overcome with patience and practice and has not caused adverse consequences in our cases.

Optic Size

Some cataract surgeons, in their zeal to minimize astigmatic effects, are moving toward smaller and smaller incision lengths, and consequently are using foldable IOLs with optics smaller than 6.0 mm. Optics of this size, even with perfect centration, can lead to bothersome edge glare in dim lighting conditions, especially in younger patients. A larger optic clearly facilitates proper evaluation of the retinal periphery, which is of particular concern in myopic patients, those with diabetic retinopathy, and those with peripheral retinal disorders. Using a larger optic is clearly advantageous for retinal examination, laser treatment, and retinal surgery.

Length

Many surgeons are using lens implants with overall loop-to-loop lengths of 12.5 mm or less. These short lengths can result in significant decentration if one or both loops are placed in the ciliary sulcus rather than in the capsular bag.

Intraocular Lens Design Selection

Owing to the large number of variables involved, any reasonable IOL design clearly has advantages and disadvantages. In today's era of efficiency and cost-consciousness, however, it is preferable to select the IOL appropriate for most cases most of the time, thereby simplifying intraoperative decision making and reducing the surgical center's inventory of IOLs.

The ultimate goal of cataract surgery is to perform the procedure offering the best visual result in the majority of cases. A three-piece, 6.0-mm optic with a diameter of 13.5 or 14.0 mm is ideal. Selecting smaller, "less-forgiving" IOLs increases the likelihood that patients will have bothersome visual distortions postoperatively. New IOL designs will undoubtedly continue to emerge; when evaluating a new IOL, be sure to identify significant clinical advantages and disadvantages.

Intraocular Lens Insertion

Rigid Lens Insertion

In inserting IOLs with rigid optics, it is important to create an incision large enough to accommodate the full diameter of the optic, so that excessive distortion of ocular tissues or tearing of wound edges does not occur. It is important to remember that scleral wounds tend to have slightly more elasticity than their more restraining corneal counterparts.

To insert a rigid lens:

1. Grasp the IOL firmly outside of the eye, using a lens inserter with broad blades that grasp the IOL in the periphery rather than across the central visual axis, such as a Clayman or a Sinskey lens inserter.
2. Carefully introduce the loop haptic into the incision by orienting it parallel to the plane of the incision.
3. Once the optic begins to enter the incision, re-orient the curved leading edge of the loop posteriorly so that the loop clears the anterior capsular edge distally and enters the capsular bag (Figure 9-3). Failure to insert the loop into the capsular bag at this point requires further manipulations later in the operation, which increase the risk of complications such as posterior capsule rupture and zonular dehiscence.
4. Direct the optic into the bag.
5. Open the lens holder and gradually withdraw it from the wound, being careful to leave the IOL in its original position. It is sometimes useful to have a second instrument, such as a Sinskey hook, to stabilize the IOL as the forceps are withdrawn.
6. Two distinct methods of placing the trailing loop into the capsular bag exist:
   a. Dial the trailing loop haptic into the bag using a Lester hook or a Sinskey hook. Place the hook into the junction of the trailing loop haptic and optic and rotate the IOL clockwise while applying gentle posterior pressure, sliding the optic and trailing loop under the anterior capsule (Figure 9-4).
   b. A Kelman-McPherson angled tying forceps may be used to grasp the trailing loop near its tip while gently pushing it 180 degrees away from the incision by pronating the wrist (Figure 9-5), allowing the so-called crotch to slip into the capsular bag (Figure 9-6). While watching the loop-optic junction, insert a second instrument, such as a Sinskey hook, through the main incision or through a side port and exert posterior pressure on the optic

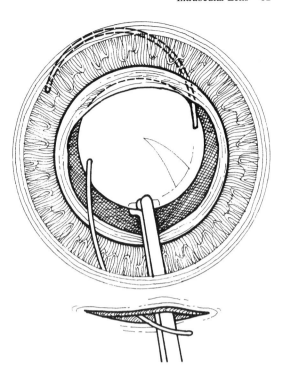

Figure 9-3. Make sure the leading loop slides posterior to the anterior capsular rim and into the capsular fornix.

near the loop, pushing the loop-optic junction under the anterior capsule (Figure 9-7). Once this is done, gently release the loop haptic, allowing the natural memory of the loop to position it into the periphery of the capsular bag.

Foldable Lens Insertion

Depending on the IOL model and manufacturer, foldable lenses are either folded manually or placed into a specially designed delivery system. Numerous IOL delivery systems are available, each with its own merits and faults, and countless others are sure to emerge as time passes. Owing to the vagaries of each system, it is critical to master techniques of IOL loading and delivery with the help of manufacturers' representatives before performing your first surgery. Even the most reliable systems are not foolproof. You should have a secondary plan and IOL in the event of an IOL problem during surgery.

Edge of anterior capsulorhexis

Figure 9-4. Dial the trailing loop into the capsular bag.

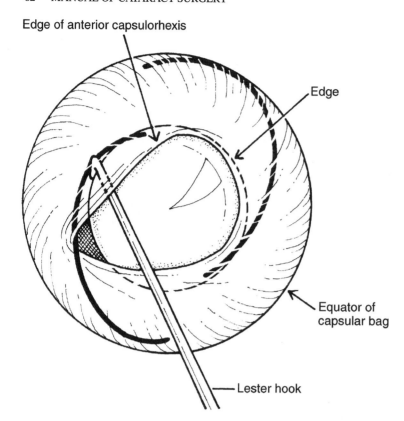

Edge

Equator of capsular bag

Lester hook

Manual Folding

Acrylic and silicone foldable lenses should be carefully folded in half according to the manufacturer's recommendations. It is important to fold the optic exactly in half, as failure to do so results in the need for a significantly longer incision. In the case of acrylic optics, the IOL may be submerged in or irrigated with warm saline to help facilitate folding and prevent cracking. In either case, acrylic foldable lenses should be folded in a very slow, smooth, and controlled fashion.

1. Grasp the folded lens with a lens inserter held parallel to the fold in the optic.
2. Introduce the lens into the incision, at first remaining parallel to the incision plane, then angling posteriorly to place the leading loop into the capsular bag.
3. Once the leading edge of the optic is posterior to the anterior capsule, supinate the right hand to bring the folded IOL perpendicular to the plane of the iris.

4. Slowly release the blades of the lens inserter and withdraw the instrument from the AC. Occasionally, a second instrument, such as a Sinskey hook, may be necessary to free the optic from the inserter.
5. Place the trailing loop into the capsular bag using either a dialing or two-handed maneuver as previously described under Intraocular Lens Insertion.

Injectable Lenses

For foldable IOLs using a delivery system:

1. Load the IOL into the cartridge according to the manufacturer's instructions, using an appropriate amount of viscoelastic. Great care should be taken to place loop haptics within the cartridge to prevent binding of the delivery mechanism, which can shear or damage the IOL.
2. Place the tip of the cartridge through the incision, gently using a forceps to raise the anterior lip of the incision if necessary. Direct the lumen of the injector toward the center of the capsular

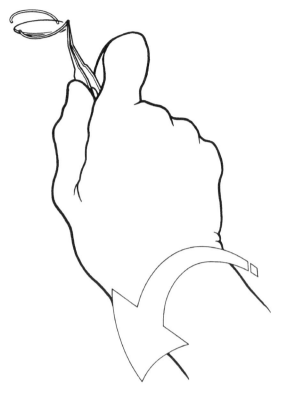

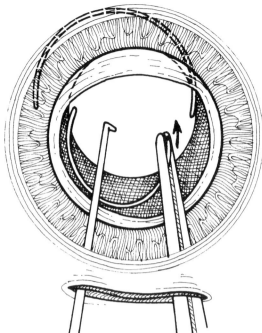

Figure 9-6. Depress posteriorly with a second instrument to ensure that the trailing loop is placed in the capsular bag and not in the ciliary sulcus.

Figure 9-5. Orientation of the trailing loop and wrist prona-tion as the loop is placed into the capsular bag.

bag, making sure the tip is slightly posterior to the plane of the anterior capsule.

3. Advance the IOL into the capsular bag using a slow, controlled motion while keeping the injec-tor stationary within the eye.

4. Once the optic is completely released, withdraw the injector without disturbing the placement of the IOL.

5. Dial or place the trailing loop as described pre-viously, or nudge the loop into the capsular bag using the delivery instrumentation, if possible.

Other Considerations

Keep in mind that an IOL may still be placed in the capsular bag even if there are radial tears in the anterior capsular rim extending to the zonular inser-tions, or if there is a discrete, circular, continuous opening in the posterior capsule.

In cases in which the capsular bag has lost struc-tural integrity, an IOL should be placed in the cil-

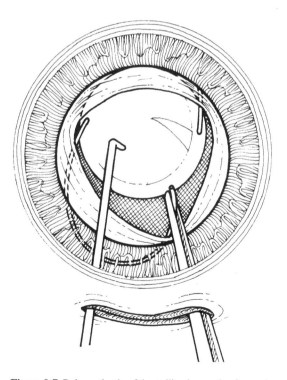

Figure 9-7. Release the tip of the trailing loop only after veri-fying that the remainder of the loop is inside the capsular bag.

iary sulcus. Loop haptics can be sufficiently supported if there are two areas of intact anterior capsular rim at least two clock-hours in size located 180 degrees apart.

As a rule, plate haptic lenses should only be placed in an intact capsular bag with a continuous anterior capsulorhexis.

With normal angles in the absence of glaucoma, an AC lens is a simple and effective choice if a posterior-chamber lens cannot be placed in the capsular bag or in the ciliary sulcus. With current AC IOL designs, the uveitis-glaucoma-hyphema (UGH) syndrome is uncommon.

In glaucoma patients, to whom conventional aqueous outflow is critical, a sutured posterior-chamber lens should be used, bearing in mind the possibilities of IOL tilt, decentration, suture erosion, and IOL dislocation.

Removal of Viscoelastic

Once the IOL is placed in a stable position with good centration, any residual viscoelastic in the AC should be removed using automated irrigation-aspiration. Failure to remove sodium hyaluronate may result in plugging of the trabecular meshwork, which can cause marked elevations in IOP. In the case of a capsular tear or a suspected capsular tear, it may be prudent to remove the viscoelastic manually using a blunt 30-gauge cannula and a 5-ml syringe. Alternatively, automated irrigation-aspiration on the lowest setting may be used to safely remove the viscoelastic in a slow, controlled fashion. The viscoelastic can often be directly visualized as it leaves the AC.

The surgeon should also give particular attention to the movement of the IOL and the movement of the posterior capsule. Quite often, especially in the case of dispersive viscoelastics, a bolus of sodium hyaluronate becomes trapped between the optic and the posterior capsule. The aspiration probe can be slipped posterior to the optic, with care taken to preserve the capsule, to remove this loculated viscoelastic. Alternatively, the probe may be used to gently tap on the optic posteriorly to squeeze the viscoelastic out from behind the IOL.

If the IOL appears to oscillate freely during irrigation-aspiration, or if there are multiple linear folds in the posterior capsule, complete removal of the viscoelastic has been accomplished. Extra care should be taken in patients with glaucomatous nerve damage to ensure the removal of all viscoelastic.

Miotics

The use of miotics at the conclusion of the case is unnecessary if the IOL is in the capsular bag and the AC is deep with a sealed wound. If an opening in the posterior capsule exists, pupillary constriction can be useful to prevent vitreous strands from moving anteriorly into the AC or to identify vitreous strands that may peak the pupillary border. If the IOL has been placed in the ciliary sulcus, and the pupil is widely dilatated, a miotic agent is recommended to prevent optic capture by the iris as it constricts postoperatively. Acetylcholine chloride (Miochol-E [CIBA Vision, Duluth, GA], 0.25 ml, 1:100) has a rapid onset and short duration of action. Alternatively, 0.01% carbachol (Miostat [Alcon, Ft. Worth, TX]), a longer-acting agent, may be used. Carbachol has both direct and indirect cholinergic properties and can be useful for its IOP-lowering effects.

Chapter 10
Wound Closure

Proper closure of a cataract incision is required to maintain structural integrity of the globe. Additionally, incision closure may have profound effects on postoperative astigmatism.

With the rising popularity of refractive surgery, patients' expectations of cataract surgery are also climbing. It is becoming more important to address refractive error when performing cataract surgery. Although accurate IOL power remains the gold standard for addressing the spheric component of the refractive error, wound construction and closure can be used to neutralize preoperative corneal astigmatism as demonstrated by corneal topography.

Nearly all properly architectured corneal and scleral wounds of reasonable size self-seal if they are constructed with care. Creating a 6.0-mm scleral tunnel wound and allowing it to self-seal without the use of sutures can result in a mild scleral shift, which can create significant corneal flattening in the incision meridian.

Sutured wound closure is indicated whenever significant wound leakage or failure to maintain a stable AC depth occurs. By adjusting the tension in the sutures, it is possible to induce a range of steepening along the incisional meridian. Suture tension is assessed subjectively, and you should come to appreciate the amount of astigmatism induced by your personal technique. Intraoperative keratometry using a simple hand-held cylindrical keratoscope is very useful in guiding suture placement and tension.

Closure of Clear Corneal Incisions

Well-constructed clear corneal incisions automatically self-seal as IOP closes the internal valve. Theoretically, the higher the IOP, the tighter the seal.

In some patients, AC shallowing occurs at the end of the surgery with clear corneal incisions. BSS through a 30-gauge round cannula should be used to hydrate the stroma at either side of the incision by wedging the tip of the cannula into the lateral extent of the incision. The clear cornea whitens as the stroma becomes hydrated, and this thickening of the stroma creates a watertight apposition of the corneal valve (Figure 10-1).

Stromal hydration should be performed judiciously and only when necessary, although the stromal edema is only temporary. Excessive hydration may result in prolonged corneal edema or even astigmatic shifts.

Closure of Scleral Tunnel Incisions

In the case of a scleral incision, corneal stromal hydration is not possible, and the wound may be reapproximated using an interrupted or a running suture if it fails to seal spontaneously. A running closure is less time consuming to place, and evenly distributes tensile forces. A series of interrupted sutures, however, allows for selective suture removal postoperatively to modulate astigmatism. Incisions constructed for the use of foldable IOLs tend to be

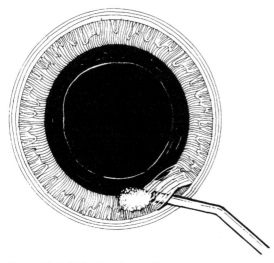

Figure 10-1. Hydration of corneal stroma.

less than 3.5 mm long and are generally closed to a watertight seal with only a single, interrupted stitch.

Placing Sutures

The most important aspect of suturing is knowing when to suture. Many surgeons are tempted to use sutures on every operation. "A stitch certainly can't hurt," they say. Be wary of this type of thinking. An improperly placed suture can most certainly do more harm than good, and this is especially true if the suture was not required in the first place.

The sutures of choice for most wounds are 9-0 or 10-0 nylon: 9-0 nylon may be particularly useful in pediatric cases, when eye rubbing may be a concern, or in cases in which 10-0 nylon "cheese-wires" through the tissues.

Three basic types of suture patterns exist: continuous, interrupted, and combined.

Continuous Sutures

To bury the knot within the incision using continuous sutures, the closure begins with the first bite through the posterior lip of the incision. The subsequent bites are placed through the anterior and posterior edges of the incision. Once bites are placed along the total length of the incision, bites are placed in the opposite direction, bisecting the distance between the previously placed suture bites (Figure 10-2). Tension is adjusted, and the suture is tied securely.

Interrupted Sutures

As with the continuous suture, the knot may be buried within the incision when using interrupted sutures by placing the bite first through only the posterior lip of the incision. Alternatively, bites may be placed across the entire wound, and the knot can be rotated and buried at the end. All interrupted sutures should be placed at the same depth, length, and suture tension to produce an even and watertight closure.

Combined Technique

In select cases with large incisions, it may be useful to use the combined technique and place both running and interrupted sutures. This combination is particularly important when there is significant tension on the wound and when selective suture removal for astigmatic control may be useful postoperatively.

Figure 10-2. Continuous running suture pattern.

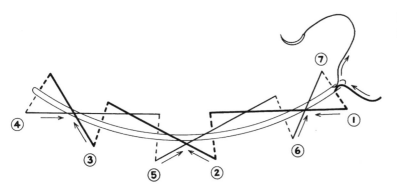

Knots

The use of a slip knot for the initial throw is recommended over triple throw for several reasons. The initial throw holds more snugly than a triple-throw, and the slip knot is amenable to adjustments in tension to help reduce postoperative astigmatic effects. The final knot tends to be more compact when using a slip knot-1-1 rather than a 3-1-1 tie.

Wound Testing

Before completing the operation, the surgeon must test the incision to verify that it is watertight. Once a cataract wound can sustain deepening of the AC thorough a side-port incision, the wound can be further stressed by applying positive pressure to the globe away from the incision site. Any incision with valve architecture can be made to leak if point pressure is applied at the incision's posterior lip. This is evidenced by the ease in expressing aqueous through a clear corneal side port less than 1 mm wide using a blunt 27-gauge cannula. With the possible exception of trauma or directed eye rubbing, few if any instances in which this type of pressure would be encountered in the standard postoperative period exist, and thus it is not clinically significant.

After removal of residual viscoelastic, BSS should be injected through a paracentesis incision. If the AC fails to deepen, a significant wound leak exists.

Intraoperative Antibiotics

Because endophthalmitis is one of the most severe and catastrophic complications of cataract surgery, measures should be taken to minimize the chances of intracameral infection.

At the conclusion of the procedure, a 0.1-ml intracameral injection of 10 mg/ml vancomycin is recommended (Gimbel, personal communication, 1998). Vancomycin is a broad-spectrum antibiotic with excellent coverage of the gram-positive organisms that are part of the normal flora of the eyelids and lashes.

The use of subconjunctival antibiotics is controversial. Subconjunctival injections are associated with their own complications, including subconjunctival hemorrhage, globe perforation, and intracameral injection. The use of topical antibiotics at the end of the operation is clearly safer than a subconjunctival injection, and if ofloxacin is used, the bioavailability of the antibiotic in the cornea and AC is excellent (Donnenfeld et al. 1997).

Removal of Lid Speculum and Drapes

Once the wound is checked, many surgeons are under the mistaken impression that the surgery is over, and they fail to pay attention to the removal of the eyelid speculum and drapes.

Atraumatic removal of the speculum is critical for avoiding corneal trauma and AC collapse. Whether a spring or self-retaining speculum is used, the blades should be first completely drawn together before attempting to disengage the eyelids. In the case of a wire speculum, one end should be firmly grasped with thumb and forefinger while the other end is squeezed toward the first using the middle finger. This method prevents the speculum from springing out of control.

When removing the drapes, take care to apply countertraction to the skin to avoid pulling the skin and subcutaneous tissues. Remember that in many cases, removal of the drapes is the most uncomfortable part of the entire procedure. Take the time and attention to do it with care.

Chapter 11
Postoperative Care

Postoperative care begins at the conclusion of the surgical procedure. At this point, the goals are to (1) prevent infection, (2) maintain normal IOP, (3) prevent an excessive inflammatory response, and (4) maximize visual function.

Postoperative Dressing

An eye patch is generally unnecessary after cataract surgery, regardless of anesthetic technique. When a regional block is used, a sturdy, perforated eye shield protects the globe from trauma, such as eye rubbing, which can lead to infection, and pressure on the eye during sleep. If the patient finds the shield uncomfortable and little risk of eye rubbing or trauma exists, the shield may be removed after a few hours after surgery as sensation returns to the eye and adnexa. In cases involving topical anesthesia, the anesthetic effect is largely gone by the time the patient leaves the recovery room and, because corneal sensation remains intact, an eye shield is not required.

Rarely, after operations involving regional anesthetic blocks, significant lagophthalmos becomes evident as the orbicularis regains function. Lagophthalmos with the potential to cause exposure keratitis should be managed with a lubricant antibiotic ointment or a pressure patch; in our experience, an ointment and shield are sufficient. Failure to take appropriate measures in the postoperative period may result in corneal trauma or keratitis sicca secondary to lagophthalmos.

Postoperative Medications

The need for postoperative antibiotics, anti-inflammatory agents, and IOP-lowering medications varies with the procedure performed and the anesthesia used.

The route of antibiotic delivery at the completion of a routine case is controversial; there are probably as many postoperative regimens as there are surgeons. The incidence of endophthalmitis is similar whether subconjunctival or topical antibiotics are used. To eliminate the risks of globe perforation and subconjunctival hemorrhage, we prefer topical agents (in addition to intracameral vancomycin, as discussed in Chapter 10). An antibiotic that covers the gram-positive organisms commonly isolated from the eyelid and conjunctival fornices should be used. Although several commercially available antibiotics exist, topical ofloxacin has been shown to have a particularly broad spectrum of coverage and excellent AC bioavailability (Donnenfeld et al. 1997). After cases in which the posterior capsule is violated (creating a potential conduit between the anterior and posterior chambers), cefazolin, vancomycin, or gentamicin, singly or in combination, may reduce the likelihood of endophthalmitis. Oral ciprofloxacin (El Baba et al. 1992) and ofloxacin (Donnenfeld et al. 1997) have been shown to attain excellent vitreal concentrations when given orally, and a 10-day postoperative course may be a reasonable alternative to intravenous medications.

A mild topical steroid or an NSAID in eyedrop form may be sufficient after an uncomplicated phacoemulsification case with a clear corneal incision. Topical rimexolone or fluorometholone should be considered in those patients with a history of elevated IOP response from prednisolone acetate (Leibowitz et al. 1996). In cases with posterior capsular openings, iris trauma, or prolonged phacoemulsification or irrigation, intravenous methylprednisolone (Solu-Medrol [Pharmacia & Upjohn Co., Bridgewater, NJ]) or dexamethasone (a longer-acting steroid) helps modulate the immune response, and a topical NSAID may decrease the incidence of postoperative uveitis and CME (Rossetti et al. 1998).

An appropriate IOP-lowering agent, such as a beta blocker, a topical carbonic anhydrase inhibitor, or an alpha$_2$-agonist, may also be used to prevent an IOP spike in the first 24 hours after surgery. Latanoprost is not recommended because of its propensity for causing CME.

Postoperative topical medications should be started on the day of surgery.

Patient Instructions

You should give patients simple, written instructions to help prevent complications and provide reassurance during the recovery period.

What to Expect after Cataract Surgery

1. After your surgery, you may experience blurred vision and minor discomfort, such as aching around your eye and numbness on the side of your face.
2. Your operated eye may not open completely until the next day. This is normal.
3. You should return to our office the day after surgery. You should also schedule other follow-up appointments over the next few weeks so we may monitor the healing process and take

measurements for any changes in your eyeglasses.
4. Please bring any eyedrops you are using in either eye to our office on each visit.

Please Do Not

1. If you receive an eye patch, *please do not* remove your eye patch. It will be removed during your first postsurgical examination.
2. *Please do not* go swimming for 1 week after your surgery.
3. *Please do not* use eye make-up for 1 week after your surgery.
4. *Please do not* rub your eyes!

Also, please be careful of small children, who may accidentally stick a finger into your operated eye.

You May

1. You may notice pink tears the first few days after your surgery. These tears are completely normal. You may use clean tissues to gently blot away drainage from around your eyes.
2. You may eat as soon as you are discharged on the day of surgery; soft foods, eaten slowly, are advisable in the first 3–4 hours.
3. You may resume any usual medications in the nonoperative eye.
4. You may take a bath or shower, shave, go to the hairdresser, or go to the barber.
5. You may sleep in any position you find comfortable.
6. You may wear tinted or clear glasses as necessary for comfort and decreased glare. If you are uncomfortable with your old glasses, please consult our office.
7. You may resume normal activities, including stooping, bending, and lifting.

If you are experiencing discomfort, take acetaminophen (Tylenol [McNeil-PPC Inc., Fort Washington, PA]) or another pain reliever. If significant discomfort persists, call our office. Most important, call the office immediately if you experience severe pain, flashing lights, or a decrease in vision.

Postoperative Follow-Up

The schedule for follow-up visits should be based on the natural history of postoperative complications. Postoperative management varies depending on the type of procedure performed and the type of anesthesia used.

Postoperative Day 1

Because wound leaks and IOP spikes may be observed within 24–36 postoperative hours, the patient should be seen the day after surgery. Assess uncorrected visual acuity to ensure that no complications resulting from surgery, including peribulbar or retrobulbar blocks, have arisen.

This examination should include the following components:

1. At a minimum, check uncorrected visual acuity and verify that it is commensurate with the examination findings.

2. Verify that the patient is compliant with the postoperative regimen of an antibiotic and anti-inflammatory.

3. Instruct the patient to call the office immediately in the event of a significant loss of vision or an increase in pain.

4. Check the integrity of the wound and the chamber depth. If significant shallowing of the AC exists, determine the cause. In the setting of low or normal IOP, check for a wound leak by checking for a Seidel sign. A significant wound leak must be repaired immediately to prevent hypotony and endophthalmitis. In the case of AC shallowing associated with high or normal IOP, consider pupillary block, aqueous misdirection syndrome (malignant glaucoma), or a choroidal hemorrhage.

5. If significant microcystic edema is noted on the first postoperative day, the IOP should be measured, as it is likely that an IOP spike has occurred. Most IOP spikes with a deep AC in the early postoperative period are secondary to retained sodium hyaluronate. The most efficacious treatment is IOP-lowering agents and the passage of time, generally a few days. Releasing fluid from the side-port incision is certainly useful for immediate IOP lowering. Unless viscoelastic is released from the AC, how-

ever, this reduction in pressure is generally temporary, often lasting less than an hour.

6. Rarely, there may be optic capture by the iris noted on the first postoperative visit. Check AC depth and the incision to rule out a wound leak. If the AC is deep and stable, instill dilating drops, position the patient in the supine position, and observe the optic. If the optic frees from the iris, instill a miotic agent, such as 2% pilocarpine. If there is persistent optic capture despite this maneuver, the IOL may require repositioning. Chronic optic capture can result in prolonged AC inflammation with synechiae formation, elevated IOP, patient discomfort, and/or CME.

The first postoperative visit can be a very positive experience for the patient. A quick, painless improvement in acuity is certainly dramatic and memorable. On the other hand, a postoperative course complicated by corneal clouding, CME, redness, irritation and tearing can leave a very negative impression of surgery despite an objective improvement in visual acuity.

Postoperative Visit Two

Because endophthalmitis most commonly presents 2–7 days after surgery (Somani et al. 1997), the patient should be examined at least once within this period to check for a decrease in vision or an increase in inflammation or pain (Lam et al. 1997). The second postoperative examination should also include testing for IOL power error and assessing the patient for an early steroid-induced IOP rise.

This examination should include:

1. Testing for best-corrected visual acuity. This allows you to verify that a lens with the correct IOL power was implanted. Any significant refractive errors caused by incorrect IOL power should be corrected at this time, when there is little or no fibrosis of the capsular bag around the IOL. Any problems associated with IOL power or position should be addressed as discussed in Chapter 14.

2. Checking IOP.

3. Careful slit-lamp examination to check for AC depth and degree of AC reaction, the presence

of any hypopyon, corneal clarity, IOL position, fibrin, keratic precipitates, posterior synechiae, and cortical or nuclear remnants. Inflammation may occur from the trauma of the procedure or from topical or intracameral agents associated with the procedure. The periorbital skin should be examined for any signs of allergy to postoperative medications.

Consider a dilated fundus examination if any suspicion of retinal breaks or retained nuclear fragments exists.

Final Postoperative Visit

The final postoperative visit is performed 2 weeks to 6 months (and sometimes longer in unusual cases) after surgery. This examination includes refraction testing and, if necessary, a new eyeglass prescription. The American Academy of Ophthalmology's Preferred Practice Patterns recommends that cataract surgery patients receive a dilated fundus examination in the operated eye within 3 months of surgery, and it is convenient to perform this the time of their final refraction testing. In our experience, asymptomatic retinal breaks or detachments after uncomplicated cataract surgery are quite rare. In the case of vitreous loss, however, a dilated fundus examination of the retinal periphery should be performed within a reasonable time to rule out tractional breaks.

The components of the final postoperative visit examination include:

1. Final refraction for distant and near vision, including a trial frame, and a prescription for glasses if indicated.
2. IOP check.
3. Dilated fundus examination to rule out retinal tears or CME, if clinically indicated.

If CME is suspected on the basis of visual acuity or biomicroscopy, consider an intravenous fluorescein angiogram to confirm or rule out the condition.

A Note on Prescribing

Historically, many optical dispensaries have convinced patients that glasses must be changed annually. The patient's desires and visual perceptions are extremely important when patients ask you if they require new glasses.

Countless patients use an old pair of glasses because they do not see as well with their new prescription. Patients become quite accustomed to the glasses they have worn for years, and unless you can offer them a substantial improvement in acuity, do not change their prescription.

Many patients undergoing sequential bilateral cataract surgery who are targeted for emmetropia require glasses only for reading. These patients may be quite comfortable with inexpensive, over-the-counter reading glasses. However, patients with significant astigmatism or symptomatic anisometropia require prescription reading glasses.

Chapter 12

The Learning Curve: Common Pitfalls during Phacoemulsification Surgery

The best way to manage an intraoperative complication is to avoid it in the first place. Although this may seem flippant, it is far easier and more effective to circumvent a difficult predicament altogether rather than try to escape it during surgery.

The following list summarizes the fundamental principles of prevention:

1. Establish realistic patient expectations at the outset. Tell patients what to expect during and after surgery.

2. Work with a cooperative and competent anesthesiologist and use adequate anesthesia and akinesia if appropriate.

3. Ensure a medically stable and cooperative patient.

4. Maximize preoperative pupillary dilatation.

5. Make sure your eyelid speculum and draping technique keeps lashes out of the operative field and allows comfortable access to the globe.

6. Take the time to position yourself and the patient comfortably.

7. Use a microscope with appropriate coaxial light and high-grade optics.

8. Reduce ambient lighting for maximum contrast.

9. Use sodium hyaluronate to assist in the procedure whenever appropriate. Never use BSS as a substitute to conserve viscoelastic, as this may damage the capsule or endothelium.

10. Master extracapsular nuclear expression before attempting phacoemulsification, so that you are comfortable if conversion from phacoemulsification to nuclear expression is necessary. Switching techniques during surgery is always challenging, but is especially difficult if you are on the early learning curve of both techniques.

11. Advance the phacoemulsifier tip steadily to emulsify rather than push the nucleus.

12. Avoid unnecessarily high phacoemulsifier power or vacuum settings.

13. Make liberal use of videotapes to refine your techniques.

14. Start with familiar techniques before making modifications. Do not try more than one new technique at a time.

15. Take courses, observe other surgeons, and ask other surgeons to observe you.

Although not often stressed, perhaps the most important fundamental principle of phacoemulsification is maintaining focus and concentration throughout the procedure. Idle conversation by support staff or visitors in the operating room should be discouraged. You must be free of distracting thoughts and concentrating solely on the task at hand; even contemplating a future step in the procedure can detract from the current step.

Managing Challenging Situations

Poor Globe Position

In cases involving topical anesthesia, the surgeon may need to ask the patient to gaze in a particular direction, depending on the step of the procedure.

The patient may be asked to look downward, for example, as the surgeon makes a superior clear corneal incision. In cases involving topical, retrobulbar, or peribulbar anesthesia, the surgeon should be aware of movements in head position. Keeping one or both hands on the patient's forehead or cheek allows surgical instruments to move in concert with unforeseen head movements.

In the event of excessive movement by the patient, surgery should be paused, and the surgeon and anesthesiologist should communicate with the patient to determine if the patient is experiencing pain, anxiety, shortness of breath, or other discomfort. Additional sedation should be administered, if indicated. If movement persists, wide (at least 1-in.) tape should be wrapped around the patient's forehead and the table's headrest to remind the patient to remain still.

If the patient squeezes his or her eyelids shut:

1. Make sure the patient is comfortable and not experiencing pain.
2. Consider supplementing the regional or topical block with local anesthetic infiltration of the orbicularis muscles.
3. Offer reassurance and remind the patient to open the eye and relax.
4. If using a wire lid speculum, switch to a self-retaining design.

Poor Visualization

Lack of clear visibility during surgery is usually obvious, but at times may be quite subtle or emerge gradually. The key is recognizing inadequate visibility. If you are having difficulty during any part of the procedure, stop and assess the quality of your view. Time and attention spent on maximizing your view is well-spent. A host of factors can impact visibility, including

1. *Lighting conditions.* Turn off overhead lights to optimize contrast. If the microscope illumination is too bright, glare or bright reflections can result. If the light is too dim, the anterior segment structures are insufficiently illuminated.

2. *Microscope light reflecting off the precorneal tear film or the corneal epithelium.* First, apply several drops of BSS onto the cornea. Tort the globe

slightly to move the reflections away from the region of interest. If too much BSS pools around the cornea, use a cellulose wick or an aspirating speculum attached to suction or a syringe to direct fluid away from the corneal surface.

3. *Instrument glare.* Use instruments with antiglare finishes whenever possible. Tort the globe or change the angle of the instrument slightly (or do both) to minimize reflection.

4. *Corneal clouding.* Check IOP by finger tension. Consider the possibility of retrobulbar hemorrhage, choroidal hemorrhage, or aqueous misdirection. Check the infusate for any compounds that may cause endothelial toxicity.

5. *Corneal striae.* Check your instrument positioning. Use your incisions and side ports as fulcrums when moving surgical instruments. The instruments should pivot at the site of the incisions rather than transmit forces anteriorly, posteriorly, or laterally at the incision site, which can result in phacoemulsifier burns or even subconjunctival blebs.

Physiologic Abnormalities

Small Pupil

Small-pupil cases are particularly challenging because the iris interferes with visibility during critical portions of surgeries, such as capsulorhexis, phacoemulsification, aspiration of residual cortex, and lens implantation. Every attempt should be made to maximize pupil size throughout preparation and the procedure itself.

It has been suggested that if there are no contraindications, patients should discontinue the use of miotic agents, such as phospholine iodide or pilocarpine, before phacoemulsification surgery. We have not found this to be of significant benefit in augmenting pupillary dilation, although it may reduce the potential inflammatory effects of miotics. Topical mydriatic eye drops should be dosed before surgery as discussed in Chapter 4. If a small pupil persists at the start of surgery, intraocular epinephrine (1:2,000) may be injected posterior to the iris to achieve further dilatation.

If these pharmacologic steps do not result in a pupil of adequate size, the pupillary margin may be stretched using two Kuglin hooks applied in

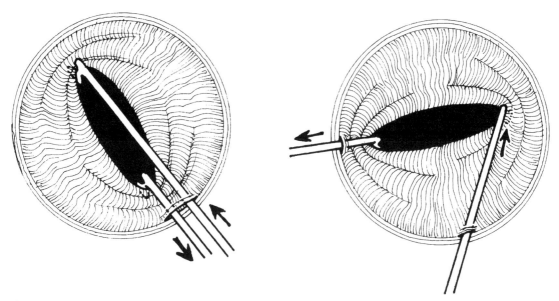

Figure 12-1. Carefully pull the hooks in opposite directions, being careful not to perforate the anterior capsule.

opposite directions. This maneuver should be repeated in the meridian 90 degrees away (Figure 12-1). With practice, this technique is fairly simple and achieves good results if the pupil is stretched for at least a few seconds. A host of mechanical devices are available for achieving pupillary dilatation, including the Beehler pupil dilator (Moria, Paris, France), which uses three retractable prongs that stretch the pupil in a manner similar to Kuglin hooks. Various iris hooks are available that stretch the pupil into a square configuration (Figure 12-2). These hooks are inserted through small, self-sealing corneal incisions. When creating openings for these hooks, angle the 15-degree blade slightly posteriorly toward the pupil, so that the resulting corneal-valve incision is in a plane directed toward the pupillary border. Although this angle mildly detracts from the sealing of the incision, it greatly facilitates hooking of the pupillary border with the iris retractors.

If mechanical methods are used to stretch the pupil, at the conclusion of the case use an intracameral miotic, such as acetylcholine or carbachol, with or without a cyclodialysis spatula to coax the pupil back into physiologic size and shape. Failure to do so may result in a chronically dilated or irregular pupil postoperatively, and this can result in severe glare disability or a decrease in visual acuity.

Hyperopia

Before the advent of viscoelastics, phacoemulsification in the hyperopic eye posed a significant challenge. Reduced axial length and shallow AC depth create a crowded working environment, and AC collapse was a constant threat. With the judicious use

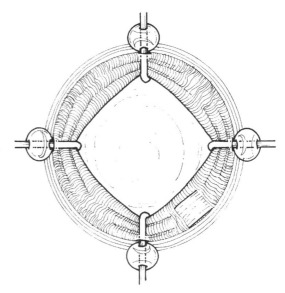

Figure 12-2. Square configuration of the pupil with iris hooks.

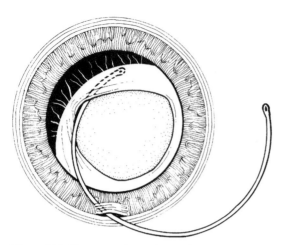

Figure 12-3. Placement of an endocapsular tension ring.

of viscoelastics, however, the hyperopic eye should not intimidate the surgeon. Surgeons who still prefer to make the eye as soft as possible before the start of the surgery may use the methods described in Chapter 4.

Zonular Abnormalities

Patients should be carefully examined preoperatively to determine the status of the lens zonules. Pseudoexfoliation, phacodonesis, or lens subluxation should be noted. If any of these conditions are present, great care should be taken throughout the surgery to minimize stress on the zonular apparatus. The capsulorhexis should be performed slowly and smoothly, as the forces used in the shearing of the capsule can result in further zonular dehiscence. Consider creating a circular anterior capsular opening with an Nd:YAG laser before taking the patient to the operating room; this prevents shearing forces on the zonules from a mechanical capsular opening. Having an Nd:YAG laser near the operating suite is indispensable.

Hydrodissection and hydrodelineation should be performed conservatively, as a quick burst of fluid into the capsular bag may create zonular tears. Phacoemulsifier power should be high enough so that the phacoemulsifier needle cuts through the nucleus easily without pushing it away. The tip should sculpt the nucleus effortlessly, without displacing the lens relative to the globe. An endocapsular tension ring or a chopping instrument may be placed inside the bag (Figure 12-3) at the equator to release cen-

tripetal forces and prevent dehisced portions of the capsular bag from being aspirated centrally (Hara et al. 1991; Gimbel at al. 1997).

A meticulous nuclear "bowling" technique, which results in inward collapse of the thinned nucleus, prevents forces from being transmitted to the zonules. An alternative method is to use phacoemulsifier chopping maneuvers, so that the mechanical force is directed entirely toward the center of the lenticular nucleus. Maneuvers, such as dividing the nucleus with a cracker or cracking the nucleus using two instruments, can also be quite effective, provided the cracking forces are directed in equal and opposite directions to prevent decentration of the capsular bag. If nuclear division techniques are used, the nucleus should be fragmented into eighths, because it is easier to draw these small wedges away from the capsular bag. Great care should be taken throughout the procedure to minimize any posteriorly directed forces, as these can cause the entire capsular bag to dislocate into the posterior chamber.

Marfan Syndrome

Characteristics of Marfan syndrome include tall stature; lanky arms and legs; a high, arched soft palate; aortic arch aneurysms; and lens dislocation, which usually occurs superotemporally. When performing cataract surgery on these patients, keep in mind that they have weak zonules of Zinn, and use the techniques outlined previously under Zonular Abnormalities. In most cases of Marfan syndrome, the patient is young, with a fairly clear, soft nucleus that can be removed primarily by high-vacuum aspiration. Nonetheless, because of the zonular collagen abnormalities found in Marfan cases, it is often impossible to retain the capsular bag, and an unintentional intracapsular cataract extraction results.

Surgical Problems

Radial Tear during Capsulorhexis

If, while performing a capsulorhexis, the tear begins to extend peripherally past the pupillary border, stop immediately. Inject viscoelastic over the radial tear, and deepen and stabilize the AC. Allowing the AC

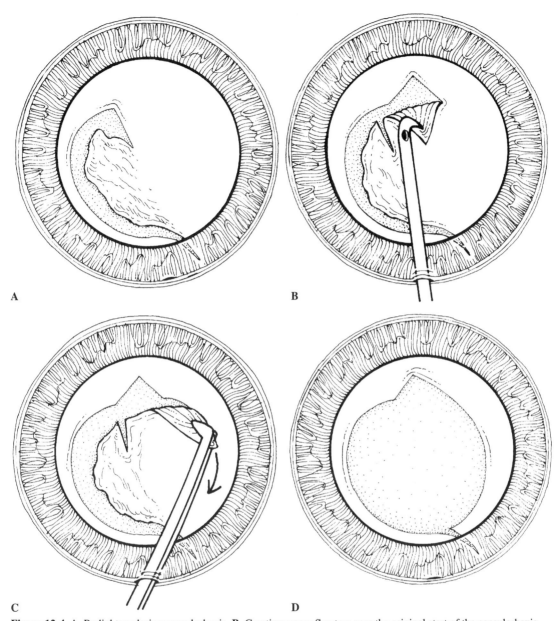

A

B

C

D

Figure 12-4. A. Radial tear during capsulorhexis. **B.** Creating a new flap tear near the original start of the capsulorhexis using a cystotome. **C.** Use forceps to guide the new tear in the opposite direction, toward the radial tear. **D.** Completed capsulorhexis in the setting of a radial tear.

to collapse may result in propagation of the tear past the lens equator, which can result in a posterior capsular rupture with an intact nucleus.

To visualize the extent of the radial tear, use a Lester or Kuglin hook to move the iris peripherally. If the leading edge of the capsulorhexis is easily seen, one hand can be used to retract the iris while the other hand continues the capsulorhexis, redirecting it centrally.

If the radial tear extends far into the periphery (i.e., to the zonular insertions or beyond) (Figure 12-4A), a new tear should be initiated on the opposite side of the rhexis. This tear is best created with a cystotome (Figure 12-4B). Using forceps to make

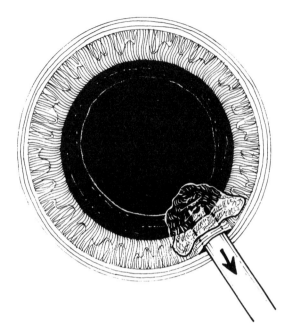

Figure 12-5. Do not use the endothelium to provide countertraction when trying to withdraw the phacoemulsifier tip from the nucleus.

the second tear is not advised, as there is little countertraction on the capsule with a pre-existing break present. Vannas scissors are very useful in creating a new flap; however, they are limited to select angles owing to their relatively fixed orientation in the incision.

A cystotome is a versatile instrument and can be used in any location. Create a new triangular flap tear, connecting one end to the start of the original capsulorhexis (see Figure 12-4B). Grasp the opposite end of the triangular flap with capsulorhexis forceps and guide the capsulorhexis in the opposite direction (Figure 12-4C), toward the edge of the radial tear (Figure 12-4D).

Burst Capsule during Hydrodissection

A posterior capsular rupture during hydrodissection is rare but memorable. The anterior capsulorhexis should be enlarged and the nucleus removed by expression. If the capsular rupture is not detected until phacoemulsification begins, which is usually the case, the nucleus may drop posteriorly from the posterior pressure of the phacoemulsifier tip and the

irrigation inflow. In this situation, a retina consultation should be obtained.

Shallowing of the Anterior Chamber

The surgeon must first identify that the AC is shallowing and then look for the cause. Possible causes include wound gape, inadequate incision seal around the phacoemulsification needle, positive vitreous pressure, pinched irrigation sleeve, leaking or disconnected irrigation tubing, a depleted BSS reservoir bottle, dehiscence of the wound, rupture of the posterior capsule, expulsive suprachoroidal hemorrhage, or failure to depress the irrigation foot switch.

Inadvertent Trauma to Anterior Segment Structures

The surgeon must maintain a high level of attentiveness throughout the procedure to avoid damaging corneal endothelium, iris, or posterior capsule, all of which can quickly result from an intracameral instrument or from nuclear fragments. Care should be taken when the phacoemulsifier tip is used in the periphery. Additionally, the plane of the ultrasonic needle should not move anterior to the iris plane, as this can quite easily damage the anterior capsule, the iris, or the corneal endothelium. The corneal endothelium must not be used for countertraction when trying to withdraw the phacoemulsifier tip from a nuclear fragment (Figure 12-5). Similarly, the corneal endothelium is not to be used as a backstop when advancing the phacoemulsifier tip into a nuclear fragment (Figure 12-6). Use of excessive aspiration flow rates or vacuum levels increases the likelihood of aspirating nontarget tissues.

If the iris is engaged in the phacoemulsification port, damage occurs in a fraction of a second, including iris stromal thinning and, possibly, damage to the iris sphincter muscle. The thinned sector of the iris can become quite wispy, which makes it even more likely to become engaged in the aspirating phacoemulsifier tip. Use a second instrument, such as a nucleus chopper, to push the damaged iris region away from the phacoemulsifier tip and into the periphery to prevent further trauma.

Figure 12-6. Do not use the endothelium as a point of resistance to advance the phacoemulsifier tip into a free nuclear fragment.

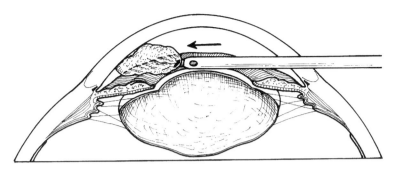

Problems with the Nucleus

Failure to Move a Nuclear Fragment Centrally

Sometimes a surgeon is unable to use the phacoemulsifier tip to draw a nuclear fragment centrally, away from the capsular fornix. This problem often results from an inadequate hydrodissection. Hydrodissection may be repeated in an effort to free remaining nuclear fragments; however, hydrodissection is often not nearly as efficacious once portions of the nucleus have been removed. The surgeon should resist the temptation to emulsify the fragment in the periphery of the capsule, where the capsular fornix, anterior capsule, posterior capsule, and iris can be easily damaged. When working in the periphery of the capsular bag, it is critical to use very short bursts of phacoemulsifier power to prevent perforating the nucleus and damaging the capsular bag.

If you are unable to draw a nuclear fragment centrally using phacoemulsifier aspiration, discontinue irrigation-aspiration, allowing the AC to shallow, which allows vitreous pressure to push the posterior capsule anteriorly. Gently use the phacoemulsifier tip as a probe and nudge the nuclear fragment centrally. Alternatively, a blunt instrument, such as a chopper or Sinskey hook, may be used for nuclear manipulation.

Managing a Posterior Plate

When nuclear cracking or chopping methods are used, incomplete nuclear fragmentation can occur if the cleavage planes do not extend all the way to the posterior nucleus. In such cases, as nuclear fragments are removed, a plate of posterior nucleus remains and rests on the posterior capsule. It can be quite difficult to engage this nuclear plate with the phacoemulsifier tip without emulsifying through to the posterior capsule.

If the residual plate is thin (Figure 12-7A), allow the AC to shallow slightly (discontinue irrigation on your phacoemulsification unit), and use a blunt second instrument to slide the plate peripherally into the capsular fornix, so that it begins to fold back onto itself (Figure 12-7B). Then engage the more accessible anterior lip of the fragment with the phacoemulsifier tip.

If the nuclear plate is rigid, insert a blunt cannula between the plate and the posterior capsule and inject viscoelastic to dissect the nuclear remnant away from the posterior capsule (Figure 12-8) to a position where it can be safely emulsified. Alternatively, a smooth second instrument, such as a Sinskey hook, can be used to gently lift one edge of the plate off of the posterior capsule and toward the phacoemulsifier tip (Figure 12-7C).

Failure to Collapse Nuclear Bowl

When using the sculpting nuclear bowl technique, minimal vacuum settings are used and the nucleus is gradually shaved away, avoiding total occlusion of the phacoemulsifier tip. The success of this technique depends on the creation of a thin nuclear "bowl" in which the remaining sides are thin enough to allow involution of the remaining nucleus. The creation of the bowl requires shaving the nucleus close to the posterior capsule without penetrating the capsule. Novice and experienced surgeons alike often make the mistake of losing their patience just as they approach the endpoint. The creation of the bowl becomes more difficult as the procedure proceeds;

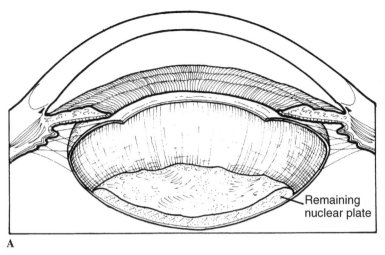

Figure 12-7. A. The posterior plate is difficult to access safely with the phacoemulsifier tip. **B.** Use the second instrument to slide the soft epinuclear shell into an accessible position. **C.** Allow the anterior chamber to shallow slightly and use a Sinskey hook to lift an edge of the nuclear plate.

A

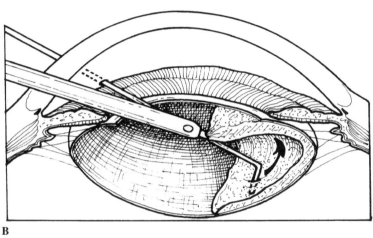

B

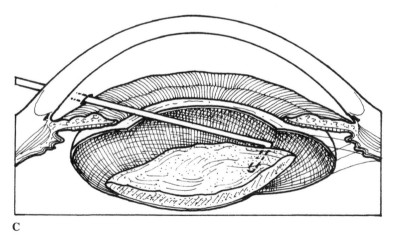

C

the initial, central sculpting demands only relatively gross movements, whereas later phacoemulsifier passes over the thin nuclear shell require very delicate movements. It is often useful to use a delicate second instrument, such as a Sinskey hook, to slide the soft nuclear shell away from the main incision, partially inverting the nuclear shell. Alternatively, if you discontinue irrigation and allow the AC to shal-

Figure 12-8. Viscodissection of the posterior plate.

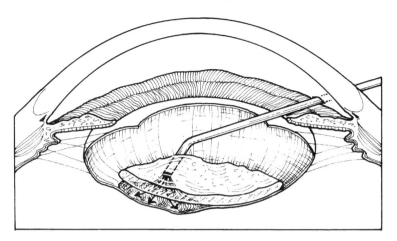

low, the phacoemulsifier tip may be used as a probe to manipulate the nuclear shell as described earlier under Failure to Move a Nuclear Fragment Centrally.

Impaled Nucleus

If, while using the one-handed technique, the surgeon finds that the phacoemulsification tip has perforated the nucleus, it may be difficult to disengage the impaled nuclear fragment from its position surrounding the tip. The cornea should not be used as a point of resistance against which the phacoemulsifier needle is withdrawn, as noted earlier under Inadvertent Trauma to Anterior Segment Structures (see Figure 12-5). In this scenario, use a second instrument to push away the nuclear fragment (Figure 12-9).

Failure to Separate Nucleus from Cortex

Sometimes, despite aggressive hydrodissection, it is still not possible to separate the nucleus from the surrounding cortex. In these cases, it is often helpful to pause and to inject viscoelastic using a blunt 30-gauge cannula into the potential plane between the lenticular nucleus and the cortex, so as to "viscodissect" the nucleus.

Inability to Visualize Peripheral Nucleus

There may be situations in which you sculpt away the central and anterior nucleus while leaving a

peripheral shell that may be hidden from view by the iris (Figure 12-10A). Attempting to "feel" the edge of the remaining nucleus without direct visualization can result in posterior capsular rupture.

A better alternative is to allow the AC to shallow slightly and use your sterile gloved thumb or forefinger to gently depress the globe near the limbus in the region of the peripheral nucleus directly opposite your incision. The pressure moves the nuclear rim into view, where it can be accessed more easily (Figure 12-10B).

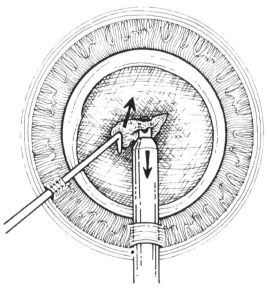

Figure 12-9. Use a second instrument to disengage the nuclear fragment, if necessary.

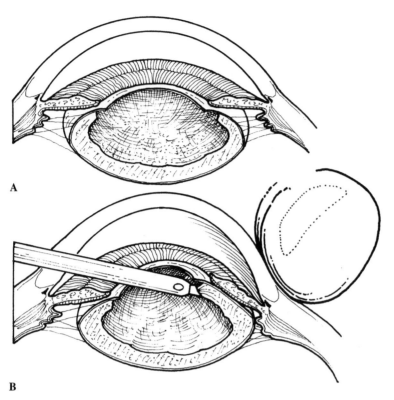

Figure 12-10. A. The anterior epinuclear shell cannot be accessed under direct visualization. **B.** Apply gentle pressure posterior to the limbus to push the epinucleus into view. Remember that the posterior capsule also moves centrally.

A

B

Circulating Nuclear Fragments

After a portion of the nucleus is removed, the remaining fragments are often freely mobile, and their sharp peripheral edges may tear the posterior capsule when circulating in the AC. Care should be taken to remove fragments from the AC in a systematic fashion to minimize the number of free-floating fragments.

Stabilization and Countertraction

Most steps during cataract surgery can be performed much more easily with the use of a second instrument to stabilize the globe. Although a 0.12 Bonn forceps is a simple and delicate instrument for countertraction, using a fixation ring provides greater stability and distributes the force over a larger area, reducing the chance of conjunctival trauma or subconjunctival hemorrhage. On the other hand, improper use of an instrument for counterpressure can result in corneal striae, a rise in IOP, and distortion of the globe.

Phacoemulsifier Burn

A number of newer, grooved phacoemulsifier sleeve designs, with channels that allow irrigation fluid to flow around the phacoemulsifier tip and cool the vibrating needle, reduce the risk of phacoemulsifier burn (Mackool 1994) (MICROFLOW, Bausch & Lomb Surgical, St. Louis, MO). Nonetheless, with dense nuclei or with tight incisions that reduce irrigation, a risk of phacoemulsifier burn still exists, which occurs when excessive ultrasound energy combined with inadequate irrigation cooling causes heat shrinkage or coagulation of corneal or scleral tissues. Phacoemulsifier burn may occur when the AC is filled with sodium hyaluronate. In this situation, viscoelastic, rather than BSS, enters the phacoemulsifier tip during aspiration, resulting in inadequate cooling of the needle.

Incision edges distorted by a phacoemulsifier burn may no longer appose in a watertight seal at the end of the procedure. Extra care must be taken to use stromal hydration with or without sutures to reapproximate the incision edges. In severe cases, a scleral patch graft may be required to close the defect, which is why it is useful to have banked scleral tissue in the operating suite at all times.

Challenges during Cortical Removal

Failure to Occlude

If the aspiration port is not fully occluded with cortex, a sufficient vacuum level does not develop and the surgeon is unable to pull cortex centrally. It is important to hold the aspiration port stationary until enough cortex occludes the tip to create a high-vacuum seal before moving it centrally. Failure to do so results in small wisps of cortex being pulled away from the capsular fornix, rather than a large confluent piece.

Inadvertently Engaging the Anterior Capsular Flap

Inadvertently engaging the anterior capsular flap is best avoided by rotating the aspirating instrument so that its port is pointing at least 20 degrees to one side, rather than directly toward the surgeon. The slight rotation of the port helps prevent the aspiration of the anterior capsule. If the capsule is actually brought into the port, this should be recognized quickly, as zonular ruptures and tears in the capsular bag can rapidly occur.

Engaging the Posterior Capsule

During the aspiration of cortex, the surgeon should be constantly watching for striae in the posterior capsule, which signal that a portion of the capsule may be in the aspiration port. Focusing the microscope at the level of the posterior capsule helps prevent this problem. If the posterior capsule becomes engaged, the microscope field suddenly reveals the puckering of the posterior capsular folds. The surgeon should recognize this condition and immediately stop aspiration. If this is done quickly enough, the posterior capsule is often still intact. If an unstable tear in the capsule results, the surgeon may wish to perform a more controlled posterior capsulorhexis to prevent the tear from being propagated peripherally.

Difficulty Removing Cortex Posterior to the Site of the Aspiration Cannula

A number of possible approaches to subincisional cortex exist, including the use of an angled irrigation-aspiration cannula or the use of bimanual irrigation-aspiration as described in Chapter 8. (See Figures 8-1 and 8-2.)

Tenacious Cortex

At times, cortex is so adherent to the surrounding capsule that standard aspiration is inadequate for its removal. A Kratz capsule scraper, a Sinskey hook, or a blunt cannula with viscodissection may be used to free the cortical material or create a flocculated surface, which may be more easily engaged by the aspiration cannula.

Residual Nuclear Fragments during Irrigation-Aspiration

During the aspiration of cortex, a previously hidden nuclear fragment sometimes appears in the AC. If this fragment is fairly small, it may be mechanically fragmented and fed into the aspirating cannula with the help of a second instrument (Figure 12-11). A large, dense nuclear fragment is best removed with the phacoemulsifier tip to avoid prolonged irrigation flow.

Detachment of Descemet's Membrane

Special care must be taken to avoid contact between intraocular instruments and the endothelium. Similarly, the surgeon must pay particular attention to Descemet's membrane while inserting instruments through the wound to avoid creating a Descemet's detachment. If stripping of Descemet's membrane occurs, the membrane should be gently replaced in its original position. If Descemet's membrane fails to adhere to its original position, the detachment

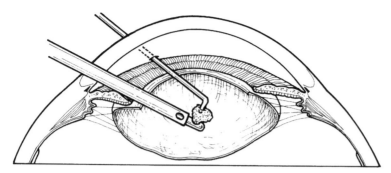

Figure 12-11. Using a Sinskey hook to feed residual nuclear fragment into irrigation-aspiration tip.

should be tamponaded with viscoelastic, air, or sulfur hexafluoride gas (SF_6) (Mahmood et al. 1998). Rarely, large detachments may require suturing.

Posterior Capsule Rupture

Perhaps the single most important aspect of managing capsular rupture is its quick detection. Failure to detect even a small opening in the posterior capsule may result in vitreoretinal traction, which can cause tearing or detachment of the retina.

Once a rent in the posterior capsule is detected, the surgeon should:

1. Stop phacoemulsification immediately and remove the phacoemulsifier needle from the eye.
2. Inject viscoelastic to stabilize the AC (ideally, simultaneously with No. 1).
3. Assess the location and extent of the tear.
4. Assess the amount of nucleus remaining.

If a posterior capsular tear occurs early in a phacoemulsification procedure, the surgeon should consider extending the wound and converting from phacoemulsification to nuclear expression to safely evacuate the lenticular nucleus.

If the opening in the posterior capsule is small, no vitreous prolapse into the AC occurs, and only a fragment of the nucleus remains, phacoemulsification may be continued with the following modifications, bearing in mind that there is an increased risk of a tractional retinal break:

1. Inject sufficient viscoelastic in the region of the capsular break to prevent anterior prolapse of vitreous strands (Figure 12-12).
2. Engage the remaining nucleus with a short burst of phacoemulsifier power, then aspirate to move the fragment anterior to the iris. A miotic may be used to prevent the nuclear fragment from dislocating posteriorly into the vitreous cavity during the remainder of phacoemulsification. Be careful to use phacoemulsifier power only when the nucleus is engaged and to use aspiration only when there is nuclear material in the port. Failure to do so results in fluid currents in the AC, which can hydrate the vitreous and cause

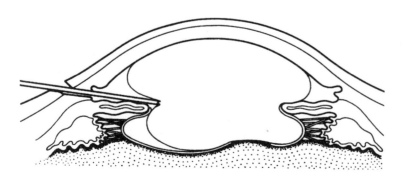

Figure 12-12. Inject viscoelastic to tamponade the posterior capsule break and prevent vitreous prolapse.

prolapse of vitreous fibers into the AC or even into the incisions.

3. Consider placing a Sheets glide through the main incision and across the pupil to prevent the posterior movement of nuclear fragments and the anterior prolapse of vitreous strands through the pupil.

After surgery, the patient should be told of an opening in the posterior capsule. Such patients often notice an abrupt increase in floaters after surgery, and this history should be elicited and addressed.

Advise the patient of the symptoms associated with retinal detachment, and perform a peripheral retinal examination postoperatively within 3 weeks to rule out an occult retinal break.

Checking for Vitreous

When an opening in the posterior capsule is recognized, check for vitreous in the AC. Rarely, there may be an intact vitreous face in the setting of a posterior capsule break, and a vitrectomy may be unnecessary.

Signs of vitreous in the AC include

1. Visible strands of vitreous.
2. Distortion of the iris caused by vitreous bands when a cyclodialysis spatula or similar instrument is swept across the pupil.
3. Nuclear fragments failing to circulate freely during phacoemulsification.
4. The appearance of a vitreous band when a methylcellulose sponge is placed at the incision and pulled slowly away from the globe. If this is noted, stop pulling immediately and transect the band using Vannas scissors (Figure 12-13).
5. Sudden deepening of the AC. This can occur if hydrated vitreous prolapses into the AC, pushing the iris posteriorly.

Anterior Vitrectomy

Despite vigilance and optimal technique, cases in which a vitrectomy is unavoidable exist.

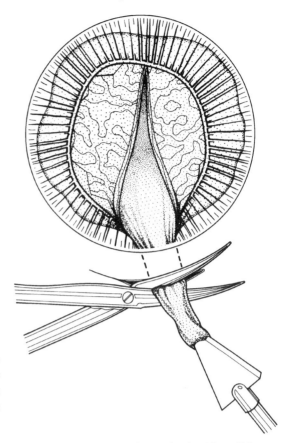

Figure 12-13. Identifying vitreous bands with a cellulose sponge.

Whenever there is a break in the posterior capsule and signs of vitreous in the AC (Figure 12-14), a vitrectomy is required. To perform a vitrectomy:

1. Remove the phacoemulsification tip from the eye.

2. Inject viscoelastic into the AC, if needed, to stabilize a posterior capsular tear before or during removal of the phacoemulsifier tip.

3. Introduce the vitrector into the AC. Select the highest cutting rate possible and use low-vacuum aspiration. It is best to use no irrigation or irrigation through a separate side port to avoid hydrating the vitreous at the vitrectomy port.

4. Keep the vitrector tip facing posteriorly, toward the vitreous, which decreases the potential for traction as vitreous is drawn toward the aspiration port.

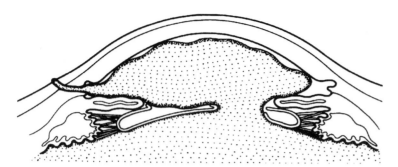

Figure 12-14. Break in posterior capsule with vitreous prolapse into anterior chamber and incision.

5. Move the vitrector slowly, being careful not to exert traction on the vitreous bands, which can cause a rhegmatogenous retinal detachment.

6. Check the wound for vitreous as described.

Always err on the side of a complete anterior vitrectomy rather than an inadequate one, as even a thin residual vitreous strand may result in CME, wound leakage, IOL decentration, or retinal detachment.

Dropped Nucleus

Despite the best surgical plans and techniques, a posterior capsular tear allowing part or all of the nucleus to dislocate posteriorly into the vitreous cavity can occur. If the nuclear fragment is very small, the patient may be followed postoperatively for signs of CME, phacoantigenic glaucoma, or retinal breaks. In the case of large nuclear fragments, a retina consultation should be obtained promptly, as a pars plana vitrectomy is indicated.

Late Retrobulbar Hemorrhage

A retrobulbar hemorrhage most commonly occurs during or soon after the administration of retrobulbar anesthesia but can occur in the middle of cataract surgery. Prompt diagnosis is the key to management. Often, the first sign is shallowing of the AC even when the bottle height is increased. Usually, a diminution of the red reflex and rise in IOP occur. If a retrobulbar hemorrhage is suspected during the case, the eye should be closed immediately. This is easily accomplished in small-incision phacoemulsification, in which the instruments are promptly removed from the eye, and the self-sealing incision and side ports close spontaneously. Observe the patient, check serial IOP measurements, and administer intravenous mannitol if necessary. If the globe softens, you may proceed with the case. If the globe remains firm, the remainder of the case must be delayed for a few days, until the IOP is normalized.

Chapter 13
Postoperative Complications

A number of potential complications after cataract surgery exist. It is not our intent to review the management of all of these situations in this manual. Serious complications, such as acute endophthalmitis and retinal detachment, should be referred to a posterior segment specialist immediately.

Cystoid Macular Edema

CME is a well-recognized complication of cataract surgery that may occur months to years after cataract surgery (Gass and Norton 1966). Risk factors for CME include diabetes, posterior capsular rupture, AC IOLs, vitreous strands to the wound, and history of CME in the fellow eye, among others. In many cases, CME is self-limited and resolves spontaneously. However, CME can become a chronic condition and may result in permanent macular damage. CME patients note a decline in vision or a failure of acuity to improve to expected levels after surgery. Determining acuity using a potential acuity meter can be quite useful to predict visual potential in CME (McDonnell et al. 1992; Sinskey and Stoppel 1994).

Treatments for CME include topical NSAIDs, such as ketorolac and diclofenac; topical steroids, such as prednisolone acetate 1% and subconjunctival injections of methylprednisolone acetate (Depo-Medrol [Pharmacia & Upjohn Co., Bridgewater, NJ]). Subconjunctival injections are preferable to injections beneath Tenon's fascia; this reduces the incidence of steroid-induced scleral melts. Although it is hard to document the effects of treatment for CME because of its high rate of spontaneous resolution, a subconjunctival steroid regimen is very effective in resistant cases. It is important to avoid prostaglandin analogs, such as latanoprost, when there is a diagnosis or risk of CME.

Subconjunctival Steroid

The technique for the administration of subconjunctival methylprednisolone acetate is as follows:

1. Instill one drop of topical 0.5% proparacaine in the conjunctival cul-de-sac.
2. Apply a 0.5% proparacaine-soaked cotton applicator to the proposed conjunctival injection site for approximately 5 minutes.
3. Using a 1-ml syringe and a 30-gauge needle, slowly insert the bevel of the needle into the subconjunctival space (Figure 13-1). Keeping the bevel toward the globe helps prevent scleral penetration.
4. The solution consists of 0.5 ml of methylprednisolone acetate (40 mg/ml) and 0.25 ml of 0.5% methylparaben-preserved bupivacaine hydrochloride, a long-acting local anesthetic. Approximately 0.5 ml of this mixture is injected.
5. Inject the solution slowly, as sudden expansion of the subconjunctival space may cause the patient discomfort.

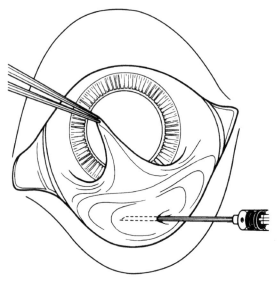

Figure 13-1. Administering a subconjunctival injection.

6. Prescribe topical prednisolone acetate 1% in conjunction with a topical NSAID.
7. Examine the patient at biweekly intervals to check corrected visual acuity and IOP.

A total of three injections may be given, one every 2 weeks (Thach et al. 1997). The first and third should be placed superotemporally, the second inferotemporally.

Propionibacterium Acnes

Propionibacterium acnes is a pleomorphic gram-positive bacillus that can cause a low-grade, indolent, postoperative endophthalmitis that may manifest as a chronic iridocyclitis. *P. acnes* infection may present several months after cataract surgery (Meisler et al. 1986). Findings are variable, but often include granulomatous keratic precipitates and white plaques within the capsular bag. It is important to keep these findings in mind when evaluating your patients several months or even years after surgery.

Chapter 14
Special Situations

Potential Corneal Problems

A number of corneal disorders that may complicate, or be aggravated by, cataract surgery exist. Use your preoperative slit-lamp examination to determine whether there is sufficient corneal disease to warrant a triple procedure (cataract extraction, IOL implantation, and penetrating keratoplasty [PK]). Endothelial cell count or corneal pachymetry may be helpful in some cases, but neither is a reliable predictor of corneal decompensation. For patients with symptomatic visual compromise resulting from both lenticular opacification and corneal clouding, plan a triple procedure to achieve visual rehabilitation. Performing sequential surgery in this setting increases costs and recovery time and subjects the patient to two separate operations. There does not appear to be a significant difference in outcome between the two approaches (Pineros et al. 1996).

Calculation of IOL Power in Triple Procedure

A triple procedure results in significant alterations of corneal curvature, AC depth, and axial length, making IOL calculation less precise than in cataract surgery alone. Numerous techniques of IOL power calculation have been described for use in triple procedures. The most accurate method of IOL calculation is the use of empirical nomograms, personalized for each physician, which relate average postoperative corneal curvature to the sizes of the donor button and the recipient bed. Alternatively, using K-readings and axial length from a normal fellow eye (if possible) can provide an excellent approximation.

Cataract Surgery with Penetrating Keratoplasty

The most significant advantage of phacoemulsification over extracapsular nuclear expression is the reduction of incision size. In a triple procedure, PK negates any potential advantages related to cataract incision size; consequently, phacoemulsification has no distinct advantage in this setting. When performing a triple procedure, use an open-sky extracapsular cataract expression in which irrigation-aspiration of cortical remnants is carried out manually using a 27-gauge cannula and 3-ml syringe (Bahadur et al. 1999).

When it is unclear whether a combined procedure is needed, inform the patient of the options and discuss the total number of operations, recovery time, anesthesia risks, and costs. A joint decision between the surgeon and patient can be made regarding the best approach for these cases.

When opting to perform phacoemulsification with IOL alone in a patient with potential endothelial compromise (i.e., without frank corneal decompensation), have a thorough discussion with the patient about the risks of subsequent corneal decompensation and the potential need for PK in the future.

Modifications in phacoemulsification technique may be required when performing cataract surgery alone. The goal is to successfully remove the cataract and insert an IOL while minimizing corneal trauma. When performing cataract extraction, special care should be taken to protect the corneal endothelium from unnecessary manipulations. As a rule, the best way for a surgeon to accomplish this is to use the phacoemulsification technique that usually works best for that particular surgeon. Many surgeons complicate these already challenging cases by changing their technique to one they think is theoretically better.

When performing the surgery, keep these principles in mind:

- Extracapsular nuclear expression is not advised in cases of corneal disease, because prolapse of the nucleus into the AC can damage the already compromised corneal endothelium. Similarly, a supracapsular approach is not appropriate in cases of endothelial compromise. A phacoemulsification procedure carefully performed in the posterior chamber is clearly preferable, as it preserves endothelial function.
- Consider using adhesive rather than cohesive viscoelastic of low to moderate molecular weight to protect the corneal endothelium. Inject the viscoelastic into the AC periodically throughout the surgery, particularly during nuclear rotation, cracking, or chopping, to maintain its protective effects on the endothelium.
- Several nuclear removal techniques may be used, including chopping, divide and conquer, and sculpting. Regardless of the approach, the goal is to prevent nuclear fragments from coming into contact with the corneal endothelium (Hayashi et al. 1996).
- Aspiration of residual cortical material after nuclear evacuation should be done judiciously, with a minimal amount of irrigation fluid. BSS PLUS Sterile Irrigating Solution (Alcon, Fort Worth, TX), which contains specialized bicarbonate buffers, glutathione, and dextrose, theoretically helps maintain endothelial cell integrity and viability.

Postoperative Management

Patients should be informed that their vision may continue to improve for up to 6 months after surgery, owing to sustained corneal edema. If corneal clarity is not documented 6 months after surgery, PK is likely indicated. During the postoperative period, patients must be reassured and counseled, as many are familiar with people without underlying corneal pathology who experience more rapid visual recovery.

Ocular inflammation should be controlled quickly with judicious use of steroids. Initial therapy, beginning on the first postoperative day, consists of topical 1% prednisolone acetate at least four times a day. These steroid drops are often used for 6 months (while monitoring IOP), and are tapered at monthly intervals to three times a day, twice a day, and once a day before they are discontinued. Five percent sodium chloride drops four times a day and 5% sodium chloride ointment at bedtime may be helpful for 3–4 weeks to treat initial postoperative corneal edema. Maintain IOP at low to normal levels postoperatively to decrease stromal edema. Any one of the variety of topical IOP-lowering agents may be used as indicated.

Pediatric Cases

Although a comprehensive discussion of the management of pediatric cataracts is beyond the scope of this text, bear in mind the following key principles.

Mature cataracts affecting the visual axis should be removed as soon as medically possible. Cortical cataracts sparing the visual axis, allowing the patient to maintain central and steady fixation, should be followed for progression. Considerable controversy exists over the minimum age required for an IOL. IOLs are being implanted successfully in patients younger than the age of 2 years, depending on the skill and experience of the surgeon (Sinskey et al. 1993b).

Many pediatric patients are unable to cooperate for an A-scan, and this often must be performed in the operating room after induction of general anesthesia. Similarly, an electronic hand-held keratometer may be required for K readings in the operating room. The IOL calculation should be performed as soon as these values are obtained so that the proper IOL can be selected immediately before the start of surgery.

Repeated administration of preoperative topical dilating drops is usually unnecessary in children and should be avoided because of possible systemic effects, particularly when using atropine, tropicamide, cyclopentolate, and phenylephrine. Depending on the medical status of the patient, intracameral epinephrine is preferable to topical phenylephrine for pupil dilation, as this minimizes systemic effects.

Because of the elastic nature of the anterior capsule and the positive intracapsular pressure from a mature, liquefied cataract, a capsulorhexis may be quite difficult to perform, and a circular capsular opening made with a vitrector is preferable (Wilson et al. 1996). Healon GV (Pharmacia & Upjohn Company, Bridgewater, NJ) may be quite helpful in small crowded eyes with an elastic sclera.

Owing to the softness of the lenticular nucleus, an irrigation-aspiration approach is used in most cases, although some exceptions require phacoemulsification. Be aware of any plaques or congenital colobomas of the posterior capsule during nuclear evacuation. A three-piece IOL with polypropylene loops is recommended for easy insertion into the small pediatric eye.

Because of the high rate of postoperative opacification of the visual axis in children (BenEzra and Cohen 1997), a primary posterior capsulotomy and anterior vitrectomy are generally recommended after IOL insertion. An alternative is to create a posterior capsulorhexis and capture the optic to prevent secondary membranes (Gimbel and DeBroff 1994).

At the conclusion of the surgery, a no-stitch valvular closure is usually impossible because of the flexibility of the sclera and cornea. Consequently, a 9-0 or 10-0 suture is generally required for wound closure. Despite the use of multiple sutures, induced astigmatism is rarely a significant problem, owing to the elasticity of the pediatric cornea and sclera.

K readings in infants change rapidly and should be replaced with average adult values in IOL calculations. A 20% undercorrection is an excellent rule of thumb for patients younger than the age of 2 years. For children between 2 and 8 years of age, a 10% undercorrection is recommended (Dahan and Drusedau 1997). The degree of myopia in adulthood can be quite variable (McClatchey and Parks 1997). The advent of successful refractive surgical procedures for adults (and more recently, even for children) makes the IOL calculation less critical than it once was.

Postoperative care should include frequent follow-up visits because of the exuberant inflammatory response characteristic of young children. It is important to instruct and supervise the child's primary caretaker to ensure effective administration of steroid, antibiotic, and cycloplegic ointments. Drops may be used, but can be difficult to administer. These medications are critical in preventing postoperative complications in children. The importance of appropriate patching to prevent amblyopia cannot be overstated.

Uveitis

First and foremost, the underlying etiology of the uveitis, if known, should be treated to reduce the occurrence of operative and postoperative complications. Ideally, the operative eye should have no signs of anterior or posterior segment inflammation for at least 4 steroid-free months before surgery. Achieving this inflammation-free interval may not always be possible, and reasonable clinical judgment must be exercised in some cases.

Patients with a history of uveitis can develop posterior synechiae, which prevent adequate pupillary dilation. Before capsulorhexis is performed, blunt dissection with a cyclodialysis spatula or Sinskey hook should be used to lyse posterior synechiae. The adhesions should be broken in a centripetal direction after the instrument is placed between the iris and the anterior capsule. In some cases, fibrotic adhesions may require sharp dissection with Vannas scissors or a bent needle. Care should be taken to avoid the liberation of excessive pigment or hemorrhage into the AC. Once adhesions along the pupillary border are lysed, iris stretching or the use of iris hooks as described in Chapter 12 may be necessary. Intravenous methylprednisolone should be used intraoperatively to minimize the effects of inflammatory mediators. Care should be taken to keep the surgery as simple as possible. Excessive or traumatic manipulations exacerbate and prolong postoperative inflammation. Pay particular attention to postoperative IOP and AC inflammation. Glaucoma secondary to prolonged topical steroid use is of significant concern in these patients.

Glaucoma and Cataracts

A number of techniques for removing cataracts in glaucoma patients exist. It is not our intent here to discuss the complex and controversial realm of glaucoma management, but rather to offer insight and help you modify your surgical technique.

In the presence of a pre-existing filtering bleb, a clear corneal cataract incision placed away from the bleb is the procedure of choice.

If a combined procedure is planned, temporal clear corneal phacoemulsification followed by a superiorly placed trabeculectomy offers excellent results (Park et al. 1997). Alternatively, the phacoemulsification may be performed superiorly through a scleral tunnel, with the same incision used for the trabeculectomy. Either approach may be used in a "non-penetrating" glaucoma procedure, as described by Robert Stegmann (Carassa et al. 1998; Stegmann et al. 1999).

Intraocular Lens Implant Complications

Advancements in surgical techniques and IOL designs, along with the advent of refractive surgery and piggyback IOLs, have greatly reduced the number of IOL revision procedures required.

Nonetheless, in a small percentage of cataract surgery cases, the IOL requires repositioning, explantation, or exchange, days or even years after surgery (Sinskey et al. 1993a). The indications for IOL repositioning or exchange include

- IOL decentration resulting in significant visual problems, such as diplopia, astigmatism, refractive changes, or disabling glare
- IOL dislocation causing symptomatic iritis, cyclitis, or UGH syndrome

Indications for IOL exchange or piggyback IOLs include those for repositioning as well as

- IOL calculation error
- Refractive result, which is unacceptable to the patient
- Miscommunication with the patient about the desired target refraction; despite detailed preoperative discussions, some patients do not appreciate the full impact of their final refractive result until after surgery
- IOL power error secondary to mislabeled IOL (this is rare)

In the case of an IOL power error, an IOL exchange or piggyback procedure should be performed within a month of surgery, before the formation of adhesions between the IOL and the lens capsule, although the exact time to fibrosis varies widely across patients and IOL designs.

Intraocular Lens Exchange

If necessary, repeat keratometry and A-scan biometry to ensure the most accurate IOL calculation. Make a reasonable attempt to obtain the model, style, power, and A-constant of the initial IOL, even if the initial surgery was performed elsewhere. Use information gained from the refractive result of the initial case to tailor your IOL power selection. For example, if the patient's result was more myopic than expected, reduce the IOL power accordingly for the new lens implant.

Explanting Specific Intraocular Lens Types

The following steps describe the technique for IOL explantation in the case of a posterior chamber IOL with loop haptics:

1. Use a YAG laser preoperatively, if necessary, to create openings in the anterior capsule, or even to transect fibrosed loop haptics. If Nd:YAG laser application is planned in the setting of a peribulbar or retrobulbar block, administer the block before the laser. If a local block is administered after Nd:YAG treatment and a retrobulbar hemorrhage occurs, precluding surgery on that day, the patient may be left with an unstable IOL. As noted in Chapter 3, having an Nd:YAG laser in close proximity to the operating room is invaluable.

2. Use a combination of corneal topography and capsule anatomy to determine incision location. Make sure the incision width is sufficient to accommodate the optic easily.

3. Keep the AC formed and deep using a generous amount of viscoelastic.

4. If there is a posterior capsular rupture, inject viscoelastic posterior to the optic for stabilization.

5. Using a blunt instrument, such as a Sinskey hook, and viscodissection, free the IOL as much as

possible from adhesions to the lens capsule. It is often useful to place two Sinskey hooks in the "crotch" (the junction between the optic and the loop) to rotate the IOL without placing asymmetric or excessive forces on the bag or zonules. If this is not possible with a reasonable amount of manipulation, amputate the loops, leave them in place, and explant the optic. Sometimes, it is then possible to go back to the loops and slide them out within their fibrotic tracts.

6. Loops may be cut with scissors or specially designed loop amputators. A pair of scissors should be specifically designated for use with haptics and IOLs, as these scissors become too dull for precise tissue cutting. When transecting loops, grasp the optic firmly with a toothed forceps or lens holder to prevent the liberated optic from dislocating posteriorly into the vitreous cavity.

7. Once the IOL or optic is removed, perform a thorough anterior vitrectomy, if necessary.

8. If sufficient capsular support exists, insert a posterior chamber IOL into the ciliary sulcus.

9. In the absence of adequate capsular support, place an AC lens or suture a posterior chamber lens into the ciliary sulcus.

Silicone Plate Haptic Intraocular Lenses

Carefully viscodissect the IOL from the capsular bag. If working through a small incision, transect the IOL in half. Several commercially available instruments designed for transecting IOLs exist. Alternatively, grasp the IOL firmly with toothed forceps and cut the IOL in half with Vannas scissors. As with loop transection, these scissors become dull when used in this manner. Once the IOL is halved, remove each fragment separately.

Anterior Chamber Intraocular Lenses with Loops

The loops of AC IOLs invariably fibrose into the angle and are difficult to mobilize. If possible, rotate the IOL, sliding the loops out of their fibrotic adhesive tracts. Otherwise, amputate the loops, remove the optic, and then slide the loops

free. If the loops cannot be removed easily, leave them in place in the angle. Follow the patient carefully postoperatively for the development of glaucoma. A vigorous attempt to remove fibrosed AC loops may result in significant iris bleeding or iridodialysis.

Early Intraocular Lens Designs

Early IOL designs include the following:

* Binkhorst 4-loop iris-supported IOLs (1960s). These IOLs were used in intracapsular procedures and are usually easy to remove owing to the absence of capsular fibrosis.
* Binkhorst 2-loop iridocapsular IOLs. If the loops of the IOLs become fibrosed, they may be transected and left in place.
* Square optics. The loops of these lenses may need to be amputated, as these lenses are not designed to rotate.
* Platinum iridium IOLs. The clip may be cut with scissors, or the loops may require amputation to free the optic.

Holes in Optics or Loops

The presence of holes in optics or loops often allows fibrosis of the capsule to take place, firmly cementing the IOL in place. These positioning holes may be used to your advantage, however, to conveniently rotate the IOL out of the bag using two Sinskey hooks and a bimanual rotation maneuver that prevents eccentric zonular forces.

Three-Piece versus One-Piece Intraocular Lenses

Owing to their intrinsic flexibility, three-piece IOLs are far easier to manipulate in exchange procedures than one-piece PMMA lenses.

Intraocular Lens Repositioning

As with an IOL exchange, the key to successful IOL repositioning is freeing the IOL from any existing capsular adhesions. Viscodissection is quite useful in this regard (Fine and Hoffman 1997).

IOL exchange or repositioning procedures are, by definition, re-operations, and often involve posterior capsular openings. Consequently, patients are prone to increased inflammatory reactions and endophthalmitis and should be carefully managed postoperatively with the appropriate use of steroids, NSAIDs, and topical and even oral antibiotics.

The Learning Curve

No two IOL exchanges or repositioning procedures are identical. Be resourceful, and be prepared to improvise your approach during each operation. Do not aimlessly insert various instruments in and out of the eye in an effort to free the initial IOL. Pause, take a minute to plan a minimally invasive strategy for your particular case, and then proceed.

Chapter 15
A Look Ahead

Cataract Surgery of the Future

Although small-incision phacoemulsification cataract surgery with topical anesthesia is an excellent technique that achieves consistent results, considerable room for improvement exists. The vibrating phacoemulsifier tip is quite effective for emulsifying the nucleus, but can rapidly damage the cornea, iris, and posterior capsule.

Laser-based systems generate far less heat than ultrasonic phacoemulsifiers, eliminating the need for irrigation fluid to cool the tip and allowing for a smaller, more streamlined probe.

A number of laser cataract-removal systems exist, including a Nd:YAG laser developed by Dr. Jack Dodick (Dodick Photolysis ARC Laser, Salt Lake City, UT, and Jona, Switzerland). Another Nd:YAG laser system, developed by Dr. Daniel Eichenbaum (Paradigm, Salt Lake City, UT), may be added as a modification to some existing phacoemulsification units. An erbium:YAG laser device (Premier Laser Systems, Irvine, CA) for cataract removal is also under development (Dodick and Bahadur 1999).

Although these laser cataract-removal techniques are currently in their infancy, they may offer the advantages of decreased incision size and greater safety. It is also conceivable that biochemical or genetic-engineering approaches to cataract management may be developed in the future.

The Perpetual Learning Curve

Everyone in the cataract surgery field, from the first-year ophthalmology resident to the experienced phacoemulsification surgeon, is on some portion of the learning curve. Although countless texts and courses on cataract surgery are available, no substitute for humility and self-criticism exists.

Perhaps the single most useful tool for self-criticism is the videotape. It is particularly important to tape and review those cases in which complications occur (even though you may be more tempted to review your stellar cases). By reviewing your difficult cases on a regular basis, preferably with the help of an experienced surgeon, you can observe your complications and errors in a relaxed environment, where you can more objectively scrutinize your movements and techniques. Many errors that were not apparent during surgery become quite clear to you after you review the case later. Without this measure of self-criticism, you are doomed to repeat the same errors repeatedly.

The realization that there is always room for improvement helps transform you from a good surgeon to an outstanding one. As you embark on the journey of self-criticism and improvement, remember to always progress in stages. Walk before you run. Do not try a new anesthesia technique, a new incision location, and a new method of nuclear disassembly all in the same operation. Change only one variable at a time. Patience is the key to successful outcomes.

References

Akahoshi T. Double Chopper Prechop. Video presentation at the Symposium on Cataract, IOL, and Refractive Surgery, Seattle, WA, June 1996.

Apple DJ, Federman JL, Krolicki TJ, et al. Irreversible silicone oil adhesion to silicone intraocular lenses: a clinicopathologic analysis. Ophthalmology 1996;103: 1555–1561, 1561–62.

Atkinson WS. Akinesia of the orbicularis. Am J Ophthalmol 1953;36:1255–1258.

Bahadur GG, Dodick JM, Gibralter RP. Phacoemulsification in Patients with Fuchs' Corneal Dystrophy. In Lu LW, Fine IH. Phacoemulsification in Difficult and Challenging Cases. New York: Thieme, 1999;41–47.

Bahadur GG, Sinskey RM. Lessons learned from IOLs. Eye World 1998;3:9–10.

BenEzra, Cohen E. Posterior capsulectomy in pediatric cataract surgery: the necessity of a choice. Ophthalmology 1997;104:2168–2174.

Carassa RG, Bettin P, Fiori M, Brancato R. Viscocanalostomy: a pilot study. Eur J Ophthalmol 1998;8:57–61.

Chehade M, Elder MJ. Intraocular lens materials and styles: a review. Aust N Z J Opththalmol 1997;25:255–263.

Cillino S, Casanova F, Cucco F, Ponte F. Topical flurbiprofen in extracapsular cataract surgery: effect on pupillary diameter and iris fluorescein leakage. J Cataract Refract Surg 1993;19:622–625.

Corbett MC, Richards AB. Intraocular adrenaline maintains mydriasis during cataract surgery. Br J Ophthalmol 1994;78:95–98.

Cuzzani OE, Ellant JP, Young PW, Gimbel HV, Rydz M. Potential acuity meter versus scanning laser ophthalmoscope to predict visual acuity in cataract patients. J Cataract Refract Surg 1998;24:263–269.

Dahan E, Drusedau MUH. Choice of lens and dioptric power in pediatric pseudophakia. J Cataract Refract Surg 1997;23:618–623.

Dodick JM, Bahadur GG. Lasers in Cataract Surgery. In LJ Singerman, G Coscas (eds), Current Techniques in Ophthalmic Laser Surgery (3rd ed). Boston: Butterworth–Heinemann, 1999;1–7.

Donnenfeld ED, Perry HD, Snyder RW, et al. Intracorneal, aqueous humor, and vitreous humor penetration of topical and oral ofloxacin. Arch Ophthalmol 1997;115: 173–176.

El Baba FZ, Trousdale MD, Gauderman WJ, et al. Intravitreal penetration of oral ciprofloxacin in humans. Ophthalmology 1992;99:483–486.

Fiore PM, Cinotti AA. Systemic effects of intraocular epinephrine during cataract surgery. Ann Ophthalmol 1988;20:23–25.

Fine IH. The chip and flip phacoemulsification technique. J Cataract Refract Surg 1991;17:366–371.

Fine IH. Cortical cleaving hydrodissection. J Cataract Refract Surg 1992;18:508–512.

Fine IH, Hoffman RS. Late reopening of fibrosed capsular bags to reposition decentered intraocular lenses. J Cataract Refract Surg 1997;23(7):990–994.

Fine IH, Maloney WF, Dillman DM. Crack and flip phacoemulsification technique. J Cataract Refract Surg 1993;19:797–802.

Flowers CW, McLeod SD, McDonnell PJ, et al. Evaluation of intraocular lens power calculation formulas in the triple procedure. J Cataract Refract Surg 1996;22: 116–122.

Gass JDM, Norton EWD. Cystoid macular edema and papilledema following cataract extraction. A fluorescein, fundoscopic, and angiographic study. Arch Ophthalmol 1966;76:646–661.

Gills JP, Cherchio M, Raanan MG. Unpreserved lidocaine to control discomfort during cataract surgery using topical anesthesia. J Cataract Refract Surg 1997;23:545–550.

Gills JP, Loyd TL. A technique of retrobulbar block with paralysis of orbicularis oculi. J Am Intraocul Implant Soc 1983;9:339–340.

Gimbel HV. Divide and conquer nucleofractis phacoemulsification: development and variations. J Cataract Refract Surg 1991;17:281–291.

Gimbel HV, DeBroff BM. Posterior capsulorhexis with optic capture: maintaining a clear visual axis after pediatric cataract surgery. J Cataract Refract Surg 1994;20: 658–664.

Gimbel HV, Kaye GB. Forceps-puncture continuous curvilinear capsulorhexis. J Cataract Refract Surg 1997;23: 473–475.

Gimbel HV, Neuhann T. Development, advantages, and methods of the continuous circular capsulorhexis technique. J Cataract Refract Surg 1990;16:31–37.

Gimbel HV, Sun R, Heston JP. Management of zonular dialysis in phacoemulsification and IOL implantation using the capsular tension ring. Ophthalmic Surg Lasers 1997;28:273–281.

Gimbel HV, Willerscheidt AB. What to do with limited view: the intumescent cataract. J Cataract Refract Surg 1993;19:657–661.

Hara T, Hara T, Yamada Y. "Equator ring" for maintenance of the completely circular contour of the capsular bag equator after cataract removal. Ophthalmic Surg 1991;22:358–359.

Hayashi K, Hayashi H, Nakao F, Hayashi F. Risk factors for corneal endothelial injury during phacoemulsification. J Cataract Refract Surg 1996;22:1079–1084.

Horiguchi M, Miyake K, Ohta I, Ito Y. Staining of the lens capsule for circular continuous capsulorhexis in eyes with white cataract. Arch Ophthalmol 1998;116:535–537.

Hsu CH, Bahadur GG, Sinskey RM. The effect of intraocular lidocaine on pupillary dilation in topical phacoemulsification. Presented at the American Society of Cataract and Refractive Surgery (ASCRS), Seattle, WA, April 12, 1999.

Jaffe NS. Cataract Surgery and Its Complications. St. Louis: Mosby, 1972.

Johansen J, Dam-Johansen M, Olson T. Contrast sensitivity with silicone and (poly)methylmethacrylate intraocular lenses. J Cataract Refract Surg 1997;23:1085–1088.

Kelman CD. Phaco-emulsification and aspiration. A new technique of cataract removal. A preliminary report. Am J Ophthalmol 1967;64:23–35.

Koch PS. Anterior chamber irrigation with unpreserved lidocaine 1% for anesthesia during cataract surgery. J Cataract Refract Surg 1997;23:551–554.

Koch PS, Katzen LE. Stop and chop phacoemulsification. J Cataract Refract Surg 1994;20:566–570.

Kohnen S, Brauweiler P. First results of cataract surgery and implantation of negative power intraocular lenses in highly myopic eyes. J Cataract Refract Surg 1996; 22:416–420.

Kohnen S, Ferrer A, Bauweiler P. Visual function in pseudophakic eyes with poly(methyl methacrylate), silicone, and acrylic intraocular lenses. J Cataract Refract Surg 1996;22:1303–1307.

Lam SR, Tuli R, Menezes A, Devenyi RG. Bacterial endophthalmitis following extracapsular cataract extraction recommendations for early detection. Can J Ophthalmol 1997;32:311–314.

Leibowitz HM, Bartlett JD, Rich R, et al. Intraocular pressure-raising potential of 1.0% rimexolone in patients responding to corticosteroids. Arch Ophthalmol 1996;114:933–977.

Mackool RJ. Preventing incision burn during phacoemulsification (letter). J Cataract Refract Surg 1994;20:357–358.

Mahmood MA, Teichmann KD, Tomey KF, et al. Detachment of Descemet's membrane. J Cataract Refract Surg 1998;24:827–833.

Maloney WF, Dillman DM, Nichamin LD. Supracapsular phacoemulsification: a capsule-free posterior chamber approach. J Cataract Refract Surg 1997;23:323–328.

Mamalis N, Phillips B, Kopp CH, et al. Neodymium:YAG capsulotomy rates after phacoemulsification with silicone posterior chamber intraocular lenses. J Cataract Refract Surg 1996;22(suppl 2):1296–1302.

McClatchey SK, Parks MM. Theoretic refractive changes after lens implantation in childhood. Ophthalmology 1997;104:1744–1751.

McDonnell PJ, Ryan SJ, Walonker AF, Miller-Scholte A. Prediction of visual acuity recovery in cystoid macular edema. Ophthalmic Surg Lasers 1992;23:354–358.

Meisler DM, Palestine AG, Vastine DW, et al. Chronic Propionibacterium endophthalmitis after extracapsular cataract extraction and intraocular lens implantation. Am J Ophthalmol 1986;102:733–739.

Mindel JS. Value of hyaluronidase in ocular surgical anesthesia. Am J Ophthalmol 1978;85:643–646.

Minkowski JS, Palese M, Guyton DL. Potential acuity meter using a minute aerial pinhole aperture. Ophthalmology 1983;90:1360–1368.

Murchison JF Jr., Shields MB. An evaluation of three surgical approaches for coexisting cataract and glaucoma. Ophthalmic Surg Lasers 1989;20:393–398.

Nadbath P, Rehman I. Facial nerve block. Am J Ophthalmol 1963;55:143–146.

Nagahara K. "Phaco-Chop," film presentation at the 3rd American-International Congress on Cataract, IOL, and Refractive Surgery, Seattle, WA, May 1993.

Nagahara K. "Phaco-chop technique eliminates central sculpting and allows faster, safer phaco." Ocular Surgery News International Edition, Oct 10, 1993;12–13.

O'Brien CS. Akinesis during cataract extraction. Arch Ophthalmol 1929;1:447–449.

Osher MS. The simple approach to intraocular lens implantation. Ophthalmic Surg Lasers 1975;6:32–35.

Oshika T, Nagata T, Ishii Y. Adhesion of lens capsule to intraocular lenses of polymethylmethacrylate, silicone, and acrylic foldable materials: an experimental study. Br J Ophthalmol 1998;82:549–553.

Park HJ, Kwon YH, Weitzman M, Caprioli J. Temporal corneal phacoemulsification in patients with filtered glaucoma. Arch Ophthalmol 1997;115:1375–1380.

Pieh S, Weghaupt H, Skorpik C. Contrast sensitivity and

glare disability with diffractive and refractive multifocal intraocular lenses. J Cataract Refract Surg 1998;24: 659–662.

Pineros OE, Cohen EJ, Rapuano CJ, Laibson PR. Triple vs. nonsimultaneous procedures in Fuch's dystrophy and cataract. Arch Ophthalmol 1996;114:525–528.

Rosenberg SE, Bahadur GG, Dodick JM. Comparison of Ultrasound Time and Power Using Chop vs. Crack Techniques for Nuclear Subdivision in Phacoemulsification. Association for Research in Vision and Ophthalmology poster presentation, 1997.

Rossetti L, Chaudhuri J, Dickersin K. Medical prophylaxis and treatment of cystoid macular edema after cataract surgery. The results of a meta-analysis. Ophthalmology 1998;105:397–405.

Schimek F, Fahle M. Techniques of facial nerve block. Br J Ophthalmol 1995;79:166–173.

Schneiderman TE, Johnson MW, Smiddy WE, et al. Surgical management of posteriorly dislocated silicone plate haptic intraocular lenses. Am J Ophthalmol 1997;123: 629–635.

Shimizu K, Misawa A, Suzuki Y. Toric intraocular lenses: correcting astigmatism while controlling axis shift. J Cataract Refract Surg 1994;20:523–526.

Sinskey RM, Amin P, Stoppel JO. Indications for and results of a large series of intraocular lens exchanges. J Cataract Refract Surg 1993a;19:68–71.

Sinskey RM, Stoppel JO. Potential acuity meter and visual outcome in pseudophakic eyes with clinical cystoid macular edema. Eur J Implant Ref Surg 1994;6:6–9.

Sinskey RM, Stoppel JO, Amin P. Long-term results of intraocular lens implantation in pediatric patients. J Cataract Refract Surg 1993b;19:405–408.

Somani S, Grinbaum A, Slomovic AR. Postoperative endophthalmitis: incidence, predisposing surgery, clinical course and outcome. Can J Ophthalmol 1997; 32:303–310.

Speaker MG, Menikoff JA. Prophylaxis of endophthalmitis with topical povidone-iodine. Ophthalmology 1991;98: 1769–1775.

Stegmann R, Pienaar A, Miller D. Visocanalostomy for open-angle glaucoma in black African patients. J Cataract Refract Surg 1999;25:316–322.

Tennen DG, Masket S. Short- and long-term effect of clear corneal incisions on intraocular pressure. J Cataract Refract Surg 1996;22:568–570.

Thach AB, Dugel PU, Flindall RJ, et al. A comparison of retrobulbar versus sub-Tenon's corticosteroid therapy for cystoid macular edema refractory to topical medications. Ophthalmology 1997;104: 2003–2008.

Van Lint H. Paralysie palpebrale temporaire provoquee par l'operation de la cataracte. Ann Ocul 1914;151:420–424.

Vaquero M, Encinas JL, Jimenez F. Visual function with monofocal versus multifocal IOLs. J Cataract Refract Surg 1996;22:1222–1225.

Vasavada AR, Desai JP. Stop, chop, chop and stuff. J Cataract Refract Surg 1996;22:526–529.

Wetchler BV. Anesthesia for Ambulatory Surgery. New York: Lippincott, 1991.

White PF. Ed. Ambulatory Anesthesia and Surgery. Philadelphia: Saunders, 1997.

Wilson ME, Saunders RA, Roberts EL, Apple DJ. Mechanized anterior capsulectomy as an alternative to manual capsulorhexis in children undergoing intraocular lens implantation. J Pediatr Ophthalmol Strabismus 1996;33:237–240.

Index

Spinal disorders, and cataract surgery, 3
Steroids, and cataract surgery, 3
    postoperative, 70
    subconjunctival administration of, 87–88
Subconjunctival hemorrhage, as complication of regional
    nerve block, 13
Superior rectus traction suture, 25
Supracapsular phacoemulsification, 50
Sutures, for wound closure, 65, 66–67
Synechiae, and cataract surgery, 5

Tobacco use, and cataract surgery, 3
Topical anesthesia, 14

Uveitis, and cataract surgery, 91

Vacuum level, setting for in nuclear evacua-
    tion, 44

Van Lint regional eyelid block, 15
Vancomycin, intracameral, 67, 69
Vasoconstrictors, for regional nerve block, 11
Videotaping of procedures, 95
Viscoelastics, for cataract surgery, 19
    removal of, 64
Visual acuity, preoperative evaluation of, 4
Visual potential, tests of, 7–8
Vitreous, preoperative evaluation of, 6

Wound closure, 65–67
    in children, 91
    for clear corneal incisions, 65
    for scleral tunnel incisions, 65–66
    sutures for, 65, 66–67
    testing of, 67

Zonular abnormalities, 76

Other Books from

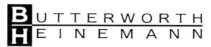

BUTTERWORTH
HEINEMANN

Atlas of Vitreous Biomicroscopy by Charles Schepens, Clement Trempe and Masataka Takahashi

1999   168pp   hb   0-7506-7052-5

Bascom Palmer Eye Institute Atlas of Ophthalmology by Richard Parrish II

1999   500pp   hb   0-7506-7075-4

1999   CD-ROM   0-7506-7076-2

Strabismus by Julio Prieto-Diaz and Carlos Souza-Diaz

1999   608pp   hb   0-7506-7129-7

Current Techniques in Ophthalmic Laser Surgery by Lawrence Singerman and Gabriel Coscas

1999   250pp   hb   0-7506-7032-0

Enucleation, Evisceration, and Exenteration of the Eye by Michael Migliori

1999   256pp   pb   0-7506-9495-5

The Pupil by Irene Loewenfeld

1999   2312pp   hb   0-7506-7143-2

Visit our web site at: www.bh.com

These books are available in bookstores or in case of difficulty call:
1-800-366-2665 in the U.S. or +44-1865-310366 in Europe.

JOIN THE BUTTERWORTH-HEINEMANN E-MAIL LIST!!!

An e-mail mailing list giving information on latest releases, special promotions, offers and other news relating to Butterworth-Heinemann titles is available. To subscribe, send an e-mail message to majordomo@world.std.com. Include in message body (not in subject line): subscribe bh-medical